UNDERSTANDING
OSTEOPOROSIS
AND ITS TREATMENT

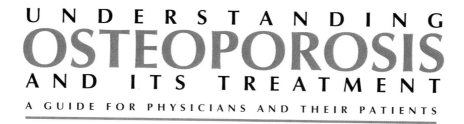

UNDERSTANDING OSTEOPOROSIS AND ITS TREATMENT

A GUIDE FOR PHYSICIANS AND THEIR PATIENTS

DR GEORGE BIRDWOOD

with a Foreword by Professor Wulf Utian

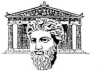

The Parthenon Publishing Group

International Publishers in Medicine, Science & Technology

NEW YORK   LONDON

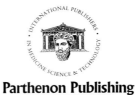

Parthenon Publishing
THE PARTHENON PUBLISHING GROUP

Published in the UK by
The Parthenon Publishing Group Limited
Casterton Hall, Carnforth, Lancs LA6 2LA, UK

Published in the USA by
The Parthenon Publishing Group Inc.
One Blue Hill Plaza, PO Box 1564, Pearl River, New York 10965, USA

Library of Congress Cataloging-in-Publication Data
Birdwood, G. F. B. (George Fortune Brodrick)
   Understanding osteoporosis and its treatment : a guide for
physicians and their patients / George Birdwood.
         p.   cm.
   Includes bibliographical references and index
   ISBN 1-85070-409-0
   1. Osteoporosis.   I. Title
   [DNLM: 1. Osteoporosis--therapy. WE 260 B618u 1995]
RC931.073B54 1995
616.716--dc20
DNLM/DLC
for Library of Congress   95-12318
                                                               CIP
                                                               Rev.

British Library Cataloguing in Publication Data
Birdwood, George
Understanding Osteoporosis and Its Treatment
   I. Title
   616.716
   ISBN 1-85070-409-0

First published in 1996

Sources of illustrations
The illustrations throughout this book are drawn from a wide variety of
different sources and reproduced with the permission of the original
copyright holders. Please see page 171 for a full listing of the permissions and sources for all the illustrations.

Designed and typeset by Rowland & Hird, Lancaster
Printed and bound in Spain by T. G. Hostench, S.A.

CONTENTS

Foreword

Osteoporosis is a word and a condition achieving increasing recognition by doctors, patients and the general public alike. Nonetheless, the number of fractures continues to escalate as the world population ages, and the cost is severe both financially and in morbidity and mortality. It was no surprise, when a North American Menopause Society/Gallup Survey was taken on women's knowledge and information sources, that only half of the menopause age respondents said their doctors had discussed their risks for osteoporosis or mechanisms for prevention[1].

A report of the Office of Technology Assessment of the Congress of the United States on hip fracture outcomes in people age 50 and over presented dramatic statistics. Hip fracture, of course, represents the most serious and costly possible outcome of osteoporosis. World-wide, an increasing number of osteoporotic hip fractures with significant morbidity and mortality can be anticipated[2]. Indeed, a World Health Organization report estimates that 30% of the world postmenopausal population meet the definition of osteoporosis and would be at substantial risk for fractures[3].

Health systems world-wide are grappling with the problem of clinical preventive services. It has been suggested that behavior and health are strongly linked. 'Improved control of behavioral risk factors, such as use of tobacco, alcohol, and other drugs, lack of exercise, and poor nutrition, could prevent half of premature deaths, one-third of all cases of acute disability, and half of all cases of chronic disability'[4].

The present monograph demonstrates a clear understanding of these issues. Under ideal circumstances, osteoporosis should be a preventable disease. Prevention of the first fracture should be a clinical goal. Dr George Birdwood has diligently researched and synthesized the subject, resulting in a clear presentation of the problem, and numerous practical guidelines to the management thereof. This book well deserves reading and studying by all health providers and receivers. While aimed at the primary physician, it would certainly be readable by all patients who have a serious and intelligent interest in their condition.

In this book, Dr Birdwood issues a strong challenge to health care providers to reduce the devastating impact of osteoporosis. I certainly hope that this challenge will be met to the benefit of us all.

Wulf H. Utian, MD, PhD
Arthur H. Bill Professor and Chairman
Department of Reproductive Biology
Case Western Reserve University School of Medicine
Director, Department of Obstetrics and Gynecology
University Hospitals of Cleveland
President, International Menopause Society

For references see page viii

References

1. Utian, W.H. and Schiff, I. (1994). NAMS Gallup Survey on Women's Knowledge, Information Sources and Attitudes to Menopause and Hormone Replacement Therapy. *Menopause*, **1**, 39–48

2. US Congress, Office of Technology Assessment, Hip Fracture Outcomes in People Age 50 and Over, Background Paper, OTA-BB-H-120, July 1994. (Washington, DC: US Government Printing Office)

3. THE WHO Study Group (1994). *Assessment of Fracture Risk and its Application to Screening for Postmenopausal Osteoporosis*. (Geneva: World Health Organization)

4. US Preventive Services Task Force (1989). *Guide to Clinical Preventive Services: An Assessment of the Effectiveness of 169 Interventions*. Report of the US Preventive Services Task Force. (Baltimore, Maryland: Williams & Wilkins)

Introduction

Lost opportunities –
the challenge of osteoporosis

Osteoporosis is commoner than most other serious diseases, but much more insidious in character. Like a thief in the night, it imperceptibly weakens the bones by slipping away with their substance. Its unwitting victims remain wholly unaware that they are losing bone, little by little, for years on end. They do not feel ill or fall sick. Their weakened bones are not diseased in themselves and produce no symptoms – until one suddenly breaks.

Only then does osteoporosis demand attention, which is often directed solely to setting the fracture it caused. The underlying bone loss which weakened the broken bone, together with other parts of the skeleton, is more likely to be overlooked than investigated and treated. Once the fracture has healed, osteoporosis may go unrecognized once again until continuing bone loss leads to further fractures, with a rising risk that they may result in death or permanent disability as the patient grows older. Sadly, that is still the natural history of osteoporosis in all too many of the postmenopausal women and old people of both sexes who are the principal cause for concern. It is also a story of lost opportunities.

Osteoporosis is the underlying cause of far more fractures than any other disease. Many of them are at major sites – the spine and neck of femur – where they carry high death rates and cause much disability, especially in the elderly. Given greater understanding of osteoporosis, many of these fractures could now be prevented, by building stronger bones in youth and controlling bone loss in susceptible adults. Recent years have seen major advances in early diagnosis and preventive treatment, which could be reducing dramatically the numbers of postmenopausal and elderly people at risk. Growing recognition of the causes of potentially serious bone loss in younger adults could also be leading to their earlier detection and treatment.

None of these measures is yet being carried out on any substantial scale. Research has given us the diagnostic and therapeutic tools required to combat osteoporosis, and clinical trials have demonstrated their efficacy, but we are not getting on with the job. The preventable is not being prevented, the diagnosable diagnosed, or the treatable treated in more than a small fraction of the many otherwise healthy people whose bones are literally dripping away, month after month, year after year. The already large numbers of fractures, disabilities and deaths attributable to osteoporosis are consequently still rising. And they are doing so even faster than the rate of increase in numbers of postmenopausal and elderly people in the population. In short, osteoporosis presents a series of challenges which are not being adequately met. As in some other fields of modern medicine, they almost all arise from failure to deliver recently developed methods of medical care when and where they are most needed. At present, we are losing the opportunity to close that gap. It should be grasped by patients and doctors alike, to prevent unnecessary bone loss before it leads to yet more fractures, and thus to even greater numbers of avoidable deaths and disabilities in the future, as the population continues to age. The key to prevention could well lie in broader understanding of osteoporosis, which this book seeks, however inadequately, to promote.

Dr George Birdwood, MA, MB, BCh
Kings Langley, England

Acknowledgements

Without Hans Dengler's original concept, this book would never have been written. Without the patience and support of Kurt Nagel, David Bloomer and Jean Wright, it might never have been brought to fruition. Without the late Dr Frank Netter's unrivalled artwork and Dr Leif Mosekilde's outstanding pictures of osteoporotic bone, it could not have been so well illustrated. The author is deeply indebted to each of them, to Jane Smalls and Monique Massotte for their work on the earlier chapters, to Dr Ivan Gillibrand and Linda Moyes for their help with additional figures, to Dr Lotte Schenkel for reviewing the proofs, and to the memory of Professor George E. Mowry for his concept of the bibliographical essay in lieu of dry reference lists. Any errors or omissions are entirely the author's own.

Further information

A range of up-to-date publications, as well as detailed information and advice for patients and professionals, is available from osteoporosis societies in many countries, notably:

The National Osteoporosis Society
PO Box 10, Radstock, Bath BA3 3YB, England

The National Osteoporosis Foundation of the USA
2100 M Street NW, Suite 602, Washington DC 20037, USA

Information about other societies can be obtained from the above or, in Europe, via The European Foundation for Osteoporosis and Bone Disease, Inserm U 234, Lyon, France.

Chapter 1:
Osteoporosis today

SOMETHING CAN BE DONE

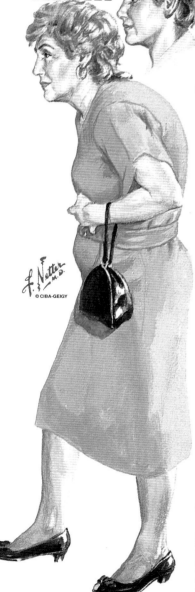

Figure 1
Thoracic kyphosis (or dowager's hump) in a postmenopausal woman, showing characteristic forward position of the head, loss of height, and abdominal protuberance – typical signs of osteoporosis, too often neglected in practice. Note contrast with youthful height and head position

Osteoporosis is not new. Old bones – and some younger ones – have long been known to break easily, but past generations simply accepted fractures in the elderly as a fact of life. It seemed quite natural that bone should become weak and brittle with age, just as the skin wrinkles and thins, muscle power wanes, and coordination falters. The skeleton could hardly be exempt from the pattern of overall decline which must always have made old people more likely to fall – and thus to fracture their increasingly fragile bones. That many of them died as a result, particularly after breaking the neck of the femur, was simply their fate. Little could be done to alter it, beyond taking granny's arm to prevent her from falling.

Two other commonplace images of osteoporosis attracted equally little critical attention in the past: the so-called 'dowager's hump', which typically rounds the upper back of women past childbearing age (*Figure 1*), and the foreshortened, often bent figures of many old people. Both have long been recorded by artists and writers. But they were simply portraying life as they saw it, not seeking to explain – still less to remedy – its infirmities. Doctors were in much the same position. Until well into this century, medicine had no power to change what fate appeared to ordain for old bones, any more than we can hinder most other aspects of aging today. There were, in any case, much greater threats to human health and well-being. When infections were still killing and disabling countless young people, and life expectancy was relatively short, the health problems of the elderly were scarcely a priority. Their fate had not yet become the challenge it presents today.

Osteoporosis itself may not be new, but it appears to be considerably more common than in the past. It is probably still on the increase, and has certainly attracted growing attention in recent years. There are several reasons for these changes. With more people in industrialized countries living longer – and breaking more bones – than ever before, osteoporosis has come to be recognized as by far the most common disorder of adult bone. The gradual bone loss which characterizes the condition is now known to underlie many more fractures, and thus to be responsible for more deaths and disability, than all other bone diseases combined. During the past decade, it has also become apparent that none of the serious consequences of osteoporosis need any longer be accepted as the inevitable fate of those most at risk – post-menopausal women and old people of both sexes – or of the rising numbers of younger victims of premature bone loss.

Stimulating the greater recognition of osteoporosis has been a growing realization that something can be done. With widespread application of modern methods of diagnosis and preventive treatment, developed in recent years, osteoporosis could now be on the decline. But nowhere have these measures yet been applied extensively enough, throughout a population at risk, to reduce the overall fracture rate. On the contrary, everywhere in the industrialized world, the total number of fractures and other consequences of osteoporotic bone loss still appear to be increasing, causing more deaths and disability with each year that passes. And that pattern will extend to many developing countries wherever living standards rise and longevity increases.

PEOPLE AT RISK

This is the challenge that osteoporosis presents today. To meet it, we must first identify those at risk. The great majority are middle-aged and older women, apparently in good health. They are, in fact, triply at risk because their skeletons are less robust than men's in the first place and are then prone to both main types of osteoporotic bone loss in succession – *postmenopausal* and *senile.*

Postmenopausal osteoporosis is caused by estrogen deficiency, irrespective of age. As its name implies, it typically affects women in their fifties and sixties, who lose bone following a normal menopause. But if ovarian production of estradiol, the female sex hormone mainly responsible for maintaining a strong skeleton, is reduced or ceases in younger women, bone loss of post-menopausal type will set in. This can happen in conjunction with persistent amenorrhea of any cause, other than pregnancy, at any age from puberty onwards. Youth gives minimal protection. In some cases, the amenorrhea may be reversible, which should prevent further deterioration but will restore little if any of the bone already lost. In others, the amenorrhea – and therefore the risk of associated bone loss – may be permanent. Removal or X-ray destruction of the ovaries (the so-called surgical menopause) or the rarer premature menopause, which inexplicably strikes some younger women, will inevitably be followed by amenorrhea and long-term bone loss, unless preventive measures are taken. Generally speaking, women of any age who are not menstruating regularly will not be secreting enough estradiol to sustain strong bones.

Although men's bones are similarly at risk if they lack the male sex hormone testosterone, its total absence is a comparatively rare event affecting well under 5% – compared with 100% of post-menopausal women. Despite talk of

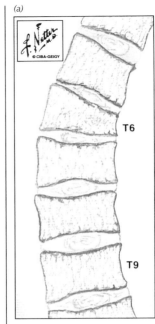
(a)

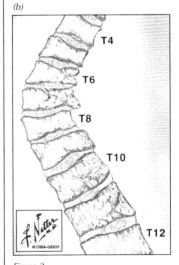
(b)

Figure 2
The underlying cause of thoracic kyphosis and the other changes seen in *Figure 1*, which typically affect postmenopausal women but also develop in a smaller number of osteoporotic men: wedging (a) and/or compression fractures (b) in the mid-thoracic vertebral bodies following years of progressive but usually symptomless bone loss

(a)

(b)

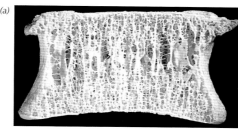
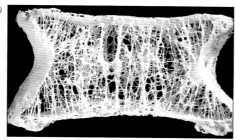

Figure 3
Osteoporosis in the lumbar spine.
The robust vertebral bodies of early
adult life (a) become rarefied after
the menopause and in old age,
losing much of their structure. (b)
They are then prone to compression
fractures – a common cause of
height loss, which may or may not
be associated with back pain

Figure 4
Common examples of fractures
in osteoporotic limb bones:
(a) intertrochanteric fracture through
lower part of femoral neck;
(b) proximal fracture of humerus;
(c) Colles' fracture of distal radius.
Wrist and arm fractures are
common in postmenopausal
women and femoral fractures in the
elderly of both sexes (see *Figure 5*)

a supposed 'male menopause', men undergo no sudden hormone withdrawal or loss of fertility in middle-age. Moreover, the few men who do lack testosterone appear to be at lower risk of osteoporosis than women deficient in estradiol, because male bones are stronger in the first place.

Estradiol deficiency makes women particularly prone to spinal osteoporosis, hence the dowager's hump, which may be its first sign. This is caused by loss of bone from the bodies of the mid-thoracic vertebrae, with risk of fracture, leading to

kyphotic curvature of the spine (*Figure 2*). Similar, sometimes more serious, changes occur in the weight-bearing bodies of the lumbar vertebrae (*Figure 3*). The vertebral bodies in otherwise healthy post-menopausal women normally lose bone quite rapidly – faster in some women than others – during the first few years after menstruation ceases. Since the bone loss itself is totally symptomless, there may be no sign of serious trouble until the bodies of one or more lumbar or thoracic vertebrae eventually collapse, often causing sudden back pain, some-times accompanied by noticeable loss of height. Victims of post-menopausal osteoporosis are also prone to bone loss and thus to fractures elsewhere (*Figure 4*). The so-called Colles' fracture just above the wrist is common in middle-aged and older women, who have usually put out an arm to save themselves from a fall, little thinking that their bones could not withstand the impact. All too often, the fracture is treated as such with little or no attention paid to the state of the bones.

Senile osteoporosis, by contrast, appears to be caused by multiple aspects of aging. These lead to progressive bone loss, somewhat different in its distribution, which afflicts the elderly of both sexes from the early to mid-seventies onwards. Ever more prone to fall as they grow older, they are increasingly at risk from hip fractures, most of them through the weakened neck (or adjacent parts) of the femur (see *Figure 4*). Even with modern surgical treatment, these fractures are still

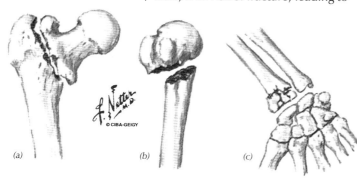

(a)

(b)

(c)

life-threatening and cause much chronic disability. Elderly women are again at greater risk from all 'osteoporotic' fractures than men of the same age (*Figure 5*). On average, they live 5–10 years longer, during which their constitutionally frailer bones, already weakened by postmenopausal osteoporosis, are increasingly – but no longer inevitably – at the mercy of the further depredations of old age (*Figure 6*).

A PECULIARLY HUMAN PROBLEM OF TODAY

The fact that most osteoporosis falls into one or other of these groups, predominantly affecting women, makes it a peculiarly human problem. Although animals can develop the disorder, its main precipitating cause, the human menopause, is unique. No other female mammal becomes infertile in this way in middle age, ceasing to produce estradiol (or other estrogens), and few species live as long. Several factors have also made osteoporosis a peculiarly late twentieth century problem. The aging of the human population in developed countries over recent decades has coincided with influences which make a growing number of young adults prone to premature bone loss. Osteoporosis is not just more recognizable, or increasing only in postmenopausal women and the elderly, but appears to be becoming more common in younger women too. These trends look set to continue well into the next century.

There are numerous factors which may already be preventing the old bones of the future from developing their full potential. Among the earliest are dietary deficiencies of calcium or vitamin D in infancy, which may continue into childhood and adolescence, and be compounded by lack of the strenuous exercise needed to stress the skeleton and build strong bones. Rapid growth at puberty requires extra calcium intake, which today's teenage diets seldom contain. If puberty is delayed for any reason, in boys or girls, lack of testosterone or estradiol will restrict both the growth and the strength of the bones. Long-term corticosteroid treatment, for asthma, arthritis or other chronic conditions, may stunt bone growth in the young as well as being a potent cause of bone loss in adults of either sex at any age. From puberty onwards, the bones may be sapped by cigarette smoking in women of childbearing age, or in either sex by excessive drinking or lack of physical exertion to maintain their strength. In young women, intensive physical training (as required by athletes and ballet dancers, for example), heroin addiction, or excessive weight loss associated with anorexia nervosa or compulsive slimming are all potential causes of amenorrhea and, therefore, of failure to build up a strong skeleton or of actual bone loss.

Figure 5
Women suffer many more vertebral, forearm and hip fractures than men, because their bones are less robust in the first place and weakened by postmenopausal bone loss before the onset of senile osteoporosis in both sexes. Note that Colles' fractures scarcely increase in men, and that hip fractures do so later than in women

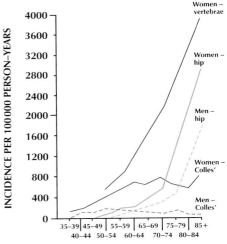

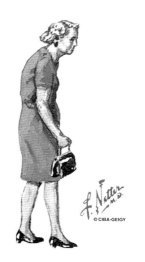

Only a small minority of the many girls identifiable in these ways are ever considered to be at risk from osteoporosis. The opportunity for timely prevention is therefore lost. The great majority will eventually enter the menopause (or old age) entirely unaware that their bones have long been in deficit. Anything that impairs bone development or subsequently promotes its loss contributes to the risk of osteoporosis later in life, because their effects are always cumulative – and bone once lost is never fully regained.

The adult human skeleton has a natural tendency to lose bone gradually, starting soon after attaining its peak mass early in adult life. If that slow loss simply continued unchanged it would not matter before the age of 100 or more. But the rate of loss tends to rise gradually in both sexes even before it is accelerated by the menopause, often by other factors as well, and ultimately by old age. None of the adverse influences which sap the bones is adequately counterbalanced, either by more favorable external factors or by the body's own feedback control mechanisms. Our bones are engaged in an unequal struggle, of which we remain sublimely unaware. Humans more than other animals, today more than in the past, some individuals more than others, and – above all – women more than men, are at increasing risk of outliving their skeletons as the population ages. Medicine has not yet fully woken up to the fact.

Figure 6
Typical images of senile osteoporosis, seldom recognized as such and still fatalistically accepted as a normal and inevitable part of growing older. Yet the symptomless bone loss which increases the risks of fracture, deformity, chronic disability and premature death can now be identified and greatly reduced

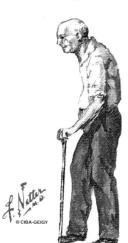

THE SCALE OF THE PROBLEM

Osteoporosis now constitutes one of the greatest health problems in industrialized countries. Its very considerable extent and severity are not receiving the necessary preventive, diagnostic or therapeutic attention. In the United Kingdom, postmenopausal women account for about one-seventh of the population – say seven million, of whom over three million will eventually suffer at least one osteoporotic fracture. At the same time, prescription records for 1991 showed that only 76 000 patients (not much more than 1% of those at risk) were receiving long-term treatment with any of the effective medications capable of preventing and/or restoring bone loss. Yet the loss of bone in osteoporosis is almost invariably progressive. If nothing is done to counter its continuing causes, notably estradiol deficiency and aging, those who have already sustained one osteoporotic fracture will be at ever-increasing risk of others. That risk could now be reduced by preventive therapy, as described in Chapter 6, and each year sees some increase in the numbers treated. But medical awareness of osteoporosis, and of the scope for its prevention, still seems to be lagging behind the opportunities opened up by recent research.

Public awareness, by contrast, has been growing rapidly with the realization that more could and should be done. In 1991, the National Osteoporosis Society in

Britain received over half a million letters seeking information and advice, and similar experiences have been reported by corresponding organizations in the USA and other industrialized countries. Women all over the developed world, from whom most enquiries come, are apparently more aware of the threat posed by osteoporosis than their doctors and more actively concerned. They have good reason to be.

THE FRACTURE RISK . . .

From the age of 50 onwards, nearly half of all white and oriental women (the risk is much lower in blacks, who have stronger bones) sustain at least one fracture of osteoporotic bone during the rest of their lives, compared with 10–15% of men. The true risks may be even higher, because the available figures quite probably underestimate the total size of the problem. Many vertebral fractures go undiagnosed, and there are few reliable statistics for wrist and other 'minor' fractures usually treated in out-patient departments. Hip fractures, by contrast, require hospital admission and, almost invariably, surgery. The figures are, therefore, recorded more reliably. They not only show how often these serious fractures occur, but also how many deaths and how much disability they precipitate.

More women now die from the after-effects of osteoporotic fractures than from all cancers of the ovaries, cervix and uterus combined. Not surprisingly, hip fracture carries the highest mortality – and the greatest risk of permanent disability. In the USA, there are over 250 000 hip fractures every year, the numbers rising with age. One woman in every four (and one in 20 men) over the age of 50 eventually fractures the neck of the femur. Most of them are over 65, many well over, an age group in which about 30% of hip fracture patients still die within 6 months, despite huge advances in pinning and other surgical techniques which aim to speed recovery and get patients rapidly on their feet again.

The elderly survivors of hip fracture do not fare well either, many failing to regain their former levels of activity and independence. Nearly half of those over 65 who recover from a fractured neck of the femur are unable to walk unaided, and nearly one-third become wholly dependent on others. Only about 20% of hip fracture patients in this age group make a full functional recovery, enabling them to resume their previous lives. To make matters worse, the total number of hip (and other) fractures in the elderly is not simply high but still growing throughout the industrialized world, at rates higher than can be explained by greater longevity alone. The increase in adverse influences on bone earlier in life could well be contributing to this trend. In the UK, there are now over 45 000 hip fractures each year, compared with only 10 000 annually in the 1960s, a rate of increase well above that of the elderly population most at risk. The number of hip fractures also rises exponentially in those over 75, and the already high risks of death, complications and/or permanent disability following fracture increase still further with advancing age.

. . . AND ITS COSTS

The social and medical costs of all this personal suffering are unacceptably high. Osteoporotic fractures not only threaten the patient's life and impair its quality. They also impose intolerable burdens on relatives or friends, often elderly themselves, and incur ever-rising expenditure on health care and supporting services as longevity increases. The health problems of the elderly are very much a priority in today's cost-conscious world.

In the United Kingdom, the hospital costs of treating osteoporotic fractures (mainly hip surgery and its aftercare) are estimated at £615 million for 1992, excluding such additional expenses as social security payments, loss of earnings, and long-term care of the disabled. In the USA, the total costs resulting from hip fractures alone were estimated to be $7200 million in 1988; they must be considerably higher today – and are bound to go on rising as people live longer, unless effective countermeasures are taken on a very substantial scale. In the United Kingdom, there are expected to be more than a million people over 85 by the end of the century, the great majority of them women at high risk of hip fracture. The proportion of postmenopausal and elderly women is already approaching one in three of the entire female population in many industrialized countries, probably exceeding that ratio in a few areas, where longevity is high and the birth rate low. Among males, about one in seven are old enough to be at risk from senile osteoporosis. No other preventable disease imperils the well-being of so many, so avoidably.

THE CASE FOR ACTION

On all these grounds, there is an overwhelming case for the early recognition and treatment of osteoporosis, and above all for its prevention. The necessary means are already at hand. It is now possible to identify the vast majority of those at high risk – though not all, because the severity of some osteoporosis is still unexplained and, therefore, unpredictable. At the same time, the sophisticated investigations now available enable bone loss to be diagnosed early, whether it was predicted or not, and the response to treatment to be monitored, both with unprecedented precision. Above all, bone loss can now be effectively controlled by the expanding range of well-tolerated drugs developed in recent years.

Hormone replacement therapy (HRT) for postmenopausal women is by far the best known, but it should now be possible to control osteoporotic bone loss in patients of either sex at any age, thus hindering or wholly preventing further deterioration and often strengthening the remaining bone to some degree.

The cost would certainly be high, but it could be justified on purely economic as well as humanitarian and social grounds. The prevention of fractures and the other costly consequences of osteoporosis should be cheaper than their treatment and aftercare.

In short, postmenopausal and (perhaps to a somewhat lesser extent) senile osteoporosis is a potentially preventable disease not actually being prevented on any appreciable scale. Only a small minority of the people with established osteoporosis are being investigated and treated today. Hardly any of those with high rates of bone loss are being identified before they become osteoporotic, and by no means all of those found to be at risk are taking effective preventive therapy.

Why should there be such a wide discrepancy between what *could* now be done to prevent bone loss and the little that is being achieved in practice? The insidious nature of osteoporosis seems to be largely responsible. It prevented the condition from being recognized in the past and still hinders its diagnosis today. Osteoporotic bone loss causes no symptoms whatever and cannot be detected by ordinary clinical examination, even with the help of routine blood tests or X-rays. The special investigations essential for a diagnosis and the most modern methods of treatment have only become generally available during the past 15 years or so. The history of osteoporosis, as we now understand it, is

consequently short, and the idea of its prevention astonishingly recent. The idea that it might be practicable to identify and treat those at high risk, as a means of preventing fractures in the elderly, was first seriously considered in the late 1970s. Only since then has osteoporosis emerged from the shadows.

OUT OF THE SHADOWS

Historically, the weak and brittle bones of the elderly received scant attention from Hippocrates and the other medical writers of antiquity. Not until the sixth century AD is there any appreciable description of a bone disease that might be osteoporosis, by Paul of Aegina, in his

Figure 7
Cortical and trabecular bone, the two distinct forms throughout the skeleton, here shown in shaft and neck of the femur, are affected differently by osteoporosis. Most osteoporotic fractures occur in predominantly trabecular bone (the neck rather than the shaft of the femur), its open framework being both weaker and more susceptible to bone loss

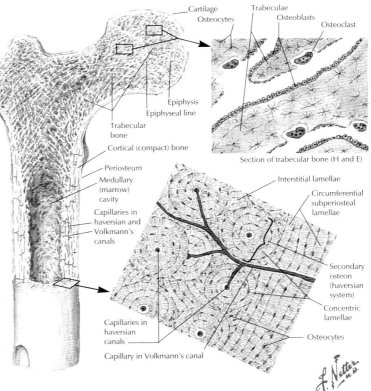

Cartilage
Osteocytes
Trabeculae
Osteoblasts
Osteoclast
Epiphysis
Epiphyseal line
Trabecular bone
Cortical (compact) bone
Periosteum
Medullary (marrow) cavity
Capillaries in haversian and Volkmann's canals
Section of trabecular bone (H and E)
Interstitial lamellae
Circumferential subperiosteal lamellae
Secondary osteon (haversian system)
Concentric lamellae
Osteocytes
Capillaries in haversian canals
Capillary in Volkmann's canal

© CIBA-GEIGY

Epitome. After that, another 1300 years of questionable references were to go by before the noted English surgeon Astley Cooper observed, in 1824, that the bones of old people became 'thin in their shell and spongy in the texture'. His description is still unrivalled for its brevity and accuracy. He seems to have been the first person to record the characteristic features of osteoporosis found in each of the two components of normal human bone, and to couple them with susceptibility to fracture, noting that the neck of the femur was vulnerable to quite modest trauma in old age.

What we now call *cortical* or compact bone, which forms the dense outer 'shell' (or cortex) of all bones and the tubular shafts of the long bones (*Figure 7*), does indeed become thinned in osteoporosis. Equally, the three-dimensional latticework of *trabecular* or cancellous bone becomes more open and spongy, eventually losing some of its internal structure (as shown in *Figure 3*). But neither Astley Cooper nor subsequent nineteenth century clinicians, who reported similar observations, if less concisely, gave a name to the condition they described. Indeed, it is questionable whether they would have regarded something with no symptoms, no recognized clinical features and no known treatment as a disease at all. It could certainly not be diagnosed in life and continued to be accepted as a normal, and therefore inevitable, effect of aging.

It was consequently left to the pathologists, early in the nineteenth century, to coin the descriptive name *osteoporosis* for the 'porous' changes they observed in the trabecular bone of the elderly. These differed from the appearances in *osteomalacia* (literally 'bone softening'), the adult counterpart of rickets in children, which was still common at the time. Both those crippling conditions had been widespread, particularly among town-dwellers, since before the industrial revolution. Crowded into slums, deprived of sunshine and malnourished, they were the relatively youthful victims of much skeletal weakness and deformity – as characteristic of their lives and times as osteoporosis is of ours today. Rickets had first been described by two London physicians in the mid-seventeenth century, and osteomalacia by a Paris surgeon 60 years later. Even then, the cause that both conditions are now known to have in common was to remain undiscovered for another 200 years.

While osteoporosis and osteomalacia both seriously impair the quality and strength of adult bone, they are now known to differ fundamentally in their nature and causation. The differences are crucial to the understanding of osteoporosis. In osteomalacia, the protein matrix which forms the framework that gives each bone its characteristic shape and structure is inadequately mineralized (*Figure 8*). In other words, the softened bones of osteomalacia contain the normal amount of structural protein but lack much of the mineral that normally makes up over two-thirds of healthy bone, giving it hardness and strength. Mineral deficiency in osteomalacia leaves the bones soft and deformable, distinguishing them from the thinned, porotic, but fully mineralized and relatively brittle bones of osteoporosis. The fact that both bone constituents, protein matrix and mineral, have been lost in proportion from osteoporotic bone means that what remains is normal in composition. The bone is not diseased but simply deficient in quantity – a fact which hindered recognition of osteoporosis in the past and still complicates its diagnosis today.

When the crucial differences between osteoporosis and osteomalacia were recognized by pathologists at the end of the last century (Table 1), they made little impact on clinicians. The first truly comprehensive textbook of general medicine, published towards the end of the nineteenth century by the renowned William Osler, makes no mention whatever of osteoporosis (or of the menopause), even in the revised editions which appeared early in the present century, though he does recommend cod-liver oil for rickets. In another textbook of the time, Dr Frederick Taylor gives a vivid account of what must have been true osteomalacia, 'beginning mostly between the ages of 30 and 40' and affecting 'women almost exclusively'. He not only gives a precise analysis of the catastrophic reduction in bone mineral content ('from 68 to 30%') but also stresses that the bones are 'so soft that they can

be cut with a knife or indented with the finger'. Cod-liver oil gets a passing mention as possible treatment, along with removal of the ovaries! Of osteoporosis there is not a word.

Not until after the First World War, when osteomalacia and rickets were already declining, thanks to better diet and living conditions, was lack of vitamin D finally identified as their cause. This discovery provided a scientific basis for their prevention, by ensuring that children and adults received adequate vitamin D, usually in the form of cod-liver oil, with exposure of the skin to sunlight. Osteoporosis continued to be the poor relation – responding little, if at all, to the new vitamin and still attracting no attention. Paradoxically, osteoporosis seems to have been cast further into obscurity when the introduction of X-rays, early in the present century, enabled

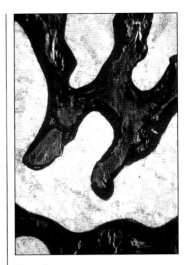

Figure 8
All bone consists of mineral deposited on a collagen framework or matrix, known as osteoid. In osteoporosis, both are reduced in proportion; there is simply too little bone of normal constitution. In osteomalacia, shown here, there is too little mineral (stained blue), as a result of vitamin D deficiency, softening the bones and leaving large areas of unmineralized osteoid (stained red)

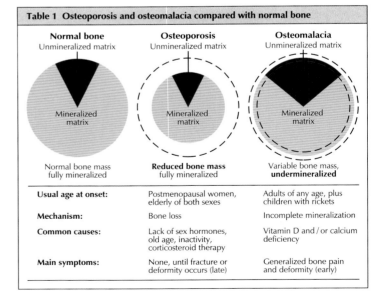

Table 1 Osteoporosis and osteomalacia compared with normal bone

	Normal bone Unmineralized matrix	**Osteoporosis** Unmineralized matrix	**Osteomalacia** Unmineralized matrix
	Mineralized matrix	Mineralized matrix	Mineralized matrix
	Normal bone mass fully mineralized	**Reduced bone mass** fully mineralized	Variable bone mass, **undermineralized**
Usual age at onset:		Postmenopausal women, elderly of both sexes	Adults of any age, plus children with rickets
Mechanism:		Bone loss	Incomplete mineralization
Common causes:		Lack of sex hormones, old age, inactivity, corticosteroid therapy	Vitamin D and / or calcium deficiency
Main symptoms:		None, until fracture or deformity occurs (late)	Generalized bone pain and deformity (early)

living bone to be visualized for the first time. X-rays could not readily distinguish between osteoporosis and osteomalacia. The bone mineral which casts X-ray shadows can be similarly deficient in both. Ordinary X-ray plates did not even enable mild-to-moderate degrees of osteoporosis to be distinguished from normal, fully mineralized bone, and despite many technical advances still do not do so (*Figure 9*). In practice, this meant that osteoporosis usually went undiagnosed until it was severe enough to have precipitated several fractures, just as it too often does today.

Right up to the Second World War, osteoporosis continued to receive more attention from the pathologists than from clinicians. As much as a third to a half of the body's total bone mass, sometimes more, was likely to have been lost before the diagnosis could be established clinically – and there was then little scope for effective treatment. Prevention was scarcely considered, for want of the necessary means to identify those most at risk or to measure or control bone loss. Little could be done, either for the few patients then thought to be osteoporotic or by the still fewer doctors who were concerned about the problem at the time.

DAWNING RECOGNITION

The crucial connection between the menopause and subsequent osteoporosis in women was made only just over 50 years ago, by Albright in 1940. By 1958, the noted Canadian

pathologist, Professor William Boyd, could write that 'Postmenopausal osteoporosis is unfortunately a very common condition, thus accounting for the frequency of fractures resulting from relatively slight trauma in elderly women.' Clinical textbooks continued to pay little attention to the condition in the 1960s and 1970s, however, some not giving it a single mention. Not until 1983 were postmenopausal and senile osteoporosis clearly distinguished and described as Types I and II, respectively, by Riggs and Melton in the USA. These surprisingly recent advances mark the beginning of our modern understanding of osteoporosis as a widespread and serious medical problem. During the past decade, its growing medical recognition has been spurred by almost annual advances in diagnostic techniques, new forms of preventive therapy, and growing evidence of their efficacy in curbing bone loss. But the greatest increase in awareness seems to have been stimulated indirectly, not by research findings or clinicians concerned about osteoporosis so much as by women's burgeoning interest in HRT – which had initially been slow to take off.

The concept attracted surprisingly little attention for several decades after estrogens were first reported to relieve hot flushes and other acute symptoms of estradiol withdrawal. This must have been partly because only about one-third of menopausal women ever have symptoms bad enough to seek relief, but mainly for several other, related reasons. The menopause, now so freely

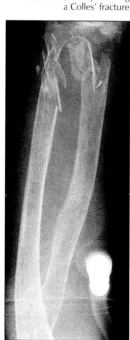

Figure 9
Although X-rays show bone much more clearly than any other tissue, they do not enable its density to be gauged with any accuracy. At least one-third of the bone mass has to be lost, most of it irretrievably, before osteoporosis can be diagnosed on an ordinary X-ray plate – in this case, clearly showing a Colles' fracture

discussed, was mentionable only in muted tones, as 'the change of life'. Its symptoms were widely regarded as being natural; many women (and most of their doctors) thought it proper to endure them, and their expectations of obtaining relief were realistically low. All this took time to change, during the first three decades after the end of the Second World War. Not until the 1980s did public interest intensify, again for several related reasons.

The long struggle for women's rights, including the right to control their own destinies in such matters as contraception and abortion, had been growing since the emancipation movement early in the century. It now burgeoned to include the menopause and HRT. Women became aware for the first time that they were destined to spend one-third or more of their lives in the estrogen-deficient postmenopausal state, which most of their grandmothers did not experience for so long and many had never reached (*Figure 10*). They also learned, mainly from women's magazines and the mass media, that something could be done to relieve hot flushes, sweats and other symptoms, such as dyspareunia, loss of libido and unpredictable mood swings, which were now becoming mentionable. Former taboos about publicly admitting the existence of the menopause (and thus of menstruation) gave way to explicit accounts of its ill effects and, above all, the liberating action of HRT, not least on a menopausal woman's sex life. Many of the middle-aged women who first tried

it already had experience of the contraceptive pill. They now began to realize, and tell their friends, that they could grasp their own destinies in another field of emancipation.

HRT STIMULATES PROGRESS

During the 1980s, demand increased for the estrogen preparations that had been under-used for several decades, most of them in tablet form but also including pessaries, ointments and subcutaneous implants. Their range was then extended, later in the decade, by the introduction of adhesive patches delivering an accurate dosage of estradiol via the skin. For the first time, HRT could really live up to its name by providing the natural hormone which is deficient after the menopause at blood levels close to those in premenopausal women. There are also sound medical reasons for preferring transdermal to oral administration, as detailed in Chapter 6. Some women preferred the skin patch to other preparations, not least because it only needed to be changed twice a week, and the media hailed it as a newsworthy novelty. By the end of the decade, more menopausal

Figure 10
Postmenopausal osteoporosis was unrecognized in the nineteenth century, when the average woman barely reached menopausal age. Despite a gradual rise of 5–10 years in the average age at menopause, increased life expectancy means that women can now expect to spend at least one-third of their lives losing bone in the estrogen-deficient, postmenopausal state – later exacerbated by senile bone loss, hence their greatly increased risk of becoming osteoporotic

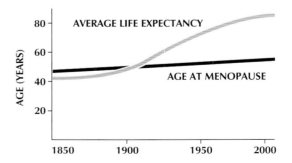

women than ever before had learned what HRT could do for their sense of well-being, their sex lives and sometimes their appearance. Only a minority were actually taking HRT, but some of them were beginning to ask whether – and, if so, why – they needed to stop taking it within a year or two, once the risk of hot flushes returning was over, and thus deprive themselves of its physical, psychological and sexual benefits. By the end of the 1980s, the psychological groundwork for long-term HRT had begun to be laid.

turned to the possible merits of long-term HRT as a prophylactic measure. It seemed to offer a possible means of combating the sustained rises, not only in osteoporosis and fractures, but also in coronary heart disease, strokes and other serious cardiovascular conditions, which normally follow the menopause (*Figure 11*). The only remaining questions were whether these common and potentially serious diseases of postmenopausal women, associated with estradiol deficiency, could be safely and effectively prevented by replacement therapy. They were answered surprisingly quickly. Clinical trials of postmenopausal women taking long-term HRT, compared with control groups receiving other active treatments or placebo, demonstrated its value in preventing bone loss within as little as 2–3 years (*Figure 12*). The very fact that the preventive effects of long-term HRT on bone loss emerged so rapidly confirmed its high efficacy, generating additional interest in osteoporosis and its prevention.

Figure 11
Estradiol appears to protect women of child-bearing age from cardiovascular disease as well as osteoporosis. Only after its withdrawal at the menopause do women (pink columns) begin to catch up with the high rates of heart attacks, strokes and other cardiovascular disorders in men

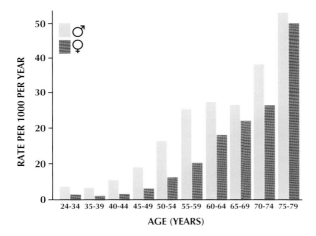

The first evidence that estrogen therapy could prevent postmenopausal osteoporosis had been published 30 years earlier – in studies showing that hormone replacement reduced height loss. Clear demonstration of reduced bone loss as such had to await the development of more accurate methods for measuring the bone density, as described in Chapter 5. By the end of the 1970s, there was no longer any doubt of the beneficial effect of estrogens, and medical attention

The estrogen component of HRT is now becoming accepted as the single most effective means (and arguably the most natural) for long-term prevention of both bone loss and cardiovascular disease in postmenopausal women. The control groups of several of the trials concerned also revealed that, without HRT, bone is lost faster than had previously been thought. In the first few years after menstruation ceases, when the body has not yet adapted to estradiol deprivation, most women lose approaching 2% of their total bone mass, and some as much as 4–5% per annum. Whatever its rate, that loss is, of course, cumulative. The total bone lost by an otherwise healthy woman of 70, following a normal menopause at say 55, may reach one-third or more of the entire skeleton she possessed 15 years earlier. She thus has to face the further ravages of senile osteoporosis with her bones already seriously depleted.

That average picture conceals much individual variation. In severe cases, the overall rate of post-menopausal bone loss can double, treble or even quadruple without obvious cause or any noticeable effects. In the bodies of the vertebrae it may reach 10% per annum in the first few postmenopausal years. In other individuals, the loss may average 1% or less, and there are no symptoms, signs or simple clinical tests to tell the fast and slow losers apart. In these respects, osteoporosis is almost as enigmatic as ever. Today, we know how to treat it preventively but are not yet able to bring the benefits of that treatment to the majority of those in need. They can be identified only by costly special investigations. Mass screening of postmenopausal women and other susceptible groups, therefore, offers the only practical prospect of early diagnosis in most of those at risk. Even this would miss some individuals, occasional men as well as women who are not ostensibly at high risk but nevertheless develop severe osteoporosis. Others will no doubt still be reluctant to accept

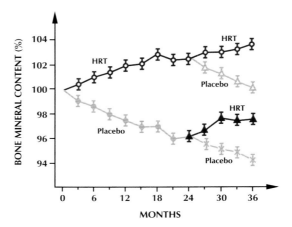

investigation or long-term treatment which they are totally unaware of needing. Greater public and professional awareness of the problem should help to overcome these hindrances and thus bring the growing scourge of osteoporosis under more adequate control in the future.

TOWARDS EFFECTIVE CONTROL

At present, osteoporosis is only just beginning to emerge from the shadows. Despite various attempts, the condition has not yet been defined in medical terms that are universally accepted. Pathologists can claim historical priority for descriptive definitions based on the bone changes they have long observed. But few clinicians (and scarcely any patients) have the opportunity to see direct evidence of such changes for themselves; reliable methods of measuring bone density have not been available for long, and they have to be repeated at intervals to estimate bone loss. Most clinical and nearly all epidemiological definitions of osteoporosis are, therefore, still based on its one unmistakable

Figure 12
A striking early demonstration that HRT prevents bone loss in recently postmenopausal women. This Danish study, published by Christiansen and colleagues in *The Lancet* in 1981, showed that an average loss of about 2% per annum from the radius in women on placebo could be converted into a net gain of over 1%, giving estrogen an overall advantage of nearly 9% after 3 years

feature: fracture. Many research studies employ fractures of the vertebral bodies and femoral neck, respectively, as criteria for post-menopausal and senile osteoporosis. The radiologists have recently been able to define osteoporosis (and measure its severity) in terms of low bone mineral content, as revealed by densitometry. But even these numerical data have to be compared with a standard representing people of the same age and sex, or set against a hypothetical peak bone mass for the individual patient, earlier in adult life. Serviceable though many of them are for particular purposes, no such definitions convey the sense of a degenerative process extending over many years. Nor do they remotely suggest the broad range of changing influences which govern that process. For the purposes of this book, osteoporosis may be quite simply defined as progressive deple-

tion of the bones, predisposing to fracture and particularly affecting postmenopausal women and the elderly.

At present, bone depletion is often advanced before it comes to light. Most patients have quite severe bone loss when they are first diagnosed, and they form only a small minority of those who need to be investigated and treated preventively. The following chapters seek to show the way forward by shedding light on the nature of normal and osteoporotic bone, and on what could now be done, both medically and by adjustment of lifestyle, to bring osteoporosis under better control. Effective prophylaxis should ideally begin with building up the skeleton to its full potential during childhood and adolescence. Even here, adverse influences may already be silently at work.

Bibliographical notes

Osteoporosis was first clearly described and so named by the Strasbourg pathologist, Jean Georges Lobstein the younger [Traité d'anatomie pathologique, Paris and Strasbourg 1829, German edition Stuttgart 1834], but there is no comprehensive account of its earlier or subsequent history. Previous references to characteristic bone loss were reported by K. Little [*Bone Behavior*, Academic Press, London and New York, 1993], while D. and C. Schapira wrote up 'Osteoporosis: The evolution of a scientific term' [Osteoporosis International (1992) 2, 164–167].

Numerous 19th century texts in French and German mention osteoporosis, usually ascribing it to loss of bone substance and to draining of its mineral salts. The latter may explain why it was not readily distinguished from the undermineralization of osteomalacia, first described by the Paris surgeon, Jean Louis Petit in 1705 [*L'art de guérir les maladies des os*. Paris, L. d'houry]. The first clear descriptions of rickets in children were earlier still [Whistler D., *Disputatio medica inauguralis, de morbo puerili Anglorum, quem patrio idiomate indigenae vocant The Rickets*. Lugduni Batavorum, ex. off. W.C.Boxii, 1645. Glisson F., De rachitide sive morbo puerili, qui vulgo The Rickets dicitur. Londini, *typ. G. Du-gardi*, 1650]. German physicians pioneered its treatment with cod-liver oil [Schütte D. (1824), Beobachtungen über den Nützen des Berger Leberthrans (Oleum jecoris Aselli, von Gadus asellus L.), *Arch. med. Erfahr.*, **2**, 79–92] and, much later, with sunlight [Huldschinsky K. (1919), Heilung von Rachitis durch künstliche Höhensonne. *Dtsch. med. Wschr.*, **45**, 712–13]. Only 3 years later, an English group showed that vitamin D promoted mineralization of bone [McCollum E.E. *et al.* (1922), Studies on experimental rickets, XXI. *J. Biol. Chem.*, **47**, 89–109].

Osteoporosis went unrecognized in almost all English and American textbooks [e.g. Osler W., *The Principles and Practice of Medicine*, 2nd edn, Young J. Pentland, Edinburgh and London, 1896; 4th edn, Henry Kimpton, London, 1901; Taylor F. *A Manual of the Practice of Medicine*, 5th edn, J. & A. Churchill, London, 1898] until well into the 20th century – and was then attributed mainly to old age. In middle-aged and younger people it remained unexplained or 'idiopathic' (literally, causing itself) until Fuller Albright *et al.* recognized estrogen deficiency as its commonest cause in 1940 [Postmenopausal osteoporosis, *Trans. Assoc. Am. Physicians*, **55**, 298–305], adding more detail in 1941 [Postmenopausal osteoporosis; its clinical features, *J. Am. Med. Assoc.*, **116**, 2465–74], and noted a promising response to estradiol, first isolated only 4 years earlier [MacCorquodale D.W. *et al.* (1936), Isolation of the principal oestrogenic substance of liquor folliculi. *J. Biol. Chem.*, **115**, 435–48].

Subsequent progress was still slow: fracture prevention was not demonstrated until over 20 years later [Gordon G.S. *et al.* (1973), Antifracture efficacy of long-term estrogens for osteoporosis, *Trans. Assoc. Am. Physicians*, **86**, 326–32], and the benefits of hormone replacement after a surgical menopause took even longer to establish [Lindsay R. *et al.* (1976), Long-term prevention of postmenopausal osteoporosis by oestrogen, *Lancet*, **i**, 1038–41]. Not until 1983 were postmenopausal and senile osteoporosis clearly distinguished [Riggs B.L. and Melton L.J., Evidence for two distinct syndromes of involutional osteoporosis, *Am. J. Med.*, **75**, 899–901]. The strikingly favorable response of postmenopausal osteoporosis to estrogen replacement had already been established in the first controlled study [Christiansen C. *et al.* (1981), Bone mass in postmenopausal women after withdrawal of oestrogen/gestagen replacement therapy, *Lancet*, **i**, 459–61].

Subsequent progress has been stimulated by development of more and more sophisticated methods of investigation (see Chapter 5), and novel forms of treatment (Chapter 6).

Chapter 2:
Normal bone and its development

A YOUTHFUL OPPORTUNITY

Osteoporosis weakens otherwise healthy bone by silently draining away its substance. To understand why the body's strongest component so often becomes dangerously wasted and brittle during the second half of life, without being diseased in

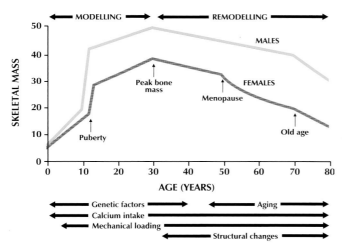

years (*Figure 1*). After that, its mass starts to decline again, very slowly at first, in both men and women, whether they eventually become significantly osteoporotic or not. That decline and the reasons why it may accelerate, sometimes becoming seriously out of control, are considered in the next chapter. This one is concerned with normal bone, with its development in youth, and with the factors which may prevent it from attaining its full potential.

The initial development of bone is a crucial phase, usually considered only in terms of growth in height. The *strength* of bone that grows normally is seldom questioned. The possibility that it might lack substance, and thus predispose to osteoporosis in later life, receives little or no attention. A unique opportunity for prevention is consequently missed. Yet girls in particular need to build up their bone mass to its full potential, to cover future outgoings. The timetable for investment is unforgiving. Only youth provides the biological opportunity to establish a substantial credit balance in the body's bone, when its natural history is still on the upswing. If that opportunity is missed, the deficit cannot be made up later in life.

Figure 1
Bone development discriminates against women long before the menopause. The peak bone mass, attained in early adulthood, is normally 30–50% higher in men. The average woman therefore has to lose only about half as much bone as a man before becoming osteoporotic – and she is likely to lose it earlier in life

itself, we must first consider normal bone: what it consists of and how it develops during childhood, adolescence and early adult life. That development does not cease when growth comes to an end, towards the end of the teens. Instead, bone continues to increase in strength, culminating in the so-called 'peak bone mass', which both sexes attain by about the age of 30. Bone then remains in its prime for only a few

The risk of osteoporosis, and its severity, does not depend simply on the rate at which bone is debited when the inevitable downswing comes, but also on the amount invested earlier. The larger the credit established in youth, the longer bone takes to become osteoporotic, whatever the cause, however fast the subsequent rate of loss. The earlier one starts to save for a pension, the less one has to curtail expenditure in retirement. The same principle applies to building up a strong skeleton, but with two major differences. The period available for investment in bone is perilously short, and the assets accumulated in youth start to drain silently away well before the age of retirement, especially in women. Prevention of osteoporosis should not be confined to belated attempts to curb this loss in the middle-aged and elderly, vital though that may be. True prophylaxis calls for a longer perspective, based on the nature of normal bone and the natural history of its development in youth.

'BONES ARE NOT STONES'

Bone is as much a living tissue as any other in the body, with a more plentiful blood supply than most and a highly active metabolism. Despite their appearance, 'bones are not stones' – in the apt words of Belgian rheumatologist, Professor Jan Dequecker. Their mineral content is high but constantly in flux, and, therefore, potentially at risk. More than two-thirds of the dry weight of the skeleton consists of the mineral hydroxyapatite (*Figure 2*), composed

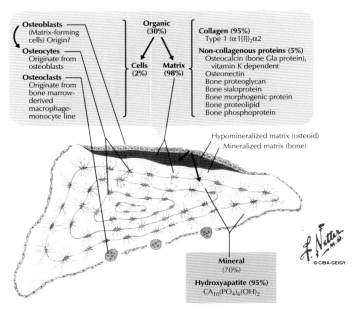

chiefly of calcium phosphate which is both supplied by and exchanged with the bloodstream. The high mineral content of normal bones gives them their stone-like hardness and weight, their rigidity and their compressive strength, but it is far from fixed or immutable, and does not provide the firm foundation on which bone is built.

What endows each bone with its characteristic shape, size and structure is the organic bone matrix. This forms the strong but flexible foundation, chiefly in the form of a specialized protein, type-I collagen, without which there would be no organized structure for the hydroxyapatite to be laid down upon. It is the collagen matrix, also known as *osteoid*, which enables bone to resist traction and torsion forces – much as the steel framework does in another calcium-rich structural mineral,

Figure 2
The composition of normal – and osteoporotic – bone. In osteoporosis the same constituents are present in the same proportions but reduced in quantity, making the bones weak and brittle. In osteomalacia, only the mineral content falls, leaving some hypomineralized matrix with consequent softening of the bones. The three cell types have distinct functions, illustrated in *Figures 3–7*

reinforced concrete. In all higher animals, collagen forms the unsung connective tissue framework which supports the characteristic structure not only of bone but of virtually all other parts of the body. It is consequently by far the most plentiful type of tissue in man and all higher animals. Without it, we should be as shapeless as jellyfish. Yet collagen, like the reinforcement in concrete, is a curiously retiring tissue, quite as inapparent in the framework of bone as it is in other tissues or organs. Together with some non-collagenous proteins (*see Figure 2*), it nevertheless makes up almost 30% of the dry matter in the human skeleton. The osteoid matrix it forms carries over twice its own weight of mineral, hydroxyapatite represent-ing about 70% of the dry weight, leaving only 0.6% of the whole for the blood vessels and cells which endow normal bone with its astonishing vitality.

The presence of so much protein in bone is as vital to its structure as the few cells and blood vessels are to its functioning as a highly responsive living tissue. Without them, bone could not grow in the first place or be constantly renewed – as it is – throughout adult life. A tissue as hard as bone can only grow by being constantly broken down and rebuilt, a process known as *modelling*. This plainly has to be highly active throughout childhood and adolescence. Perhaps more surprisingly, bone continues to be *remodelled* (*Figure 3*) not just into adult life and up to the attainment of peak bone mass, but in regular cycles right through to extreme old age. Even osteoporotic bone is continuously renewed in the same way. Indeed, it is a slight but persistent imbalance between the normal processes of breaking down and rebuilding bone which results in its gradual loss, and eventually gives rise to all forms of osteoporosis.

Figure 3
Bone is continuously renovated by remodelling, which is also the mechanism of bone loss in osteoporosis. At this remodelling site in trabecular bone (a), the large cells are osteoclasts resorbing old bone, which the many smaller osteoblasts will then replace with new, as shown in diagram (b). During growth, new bone formation exceeds resorption. In osteoporosis, it fails to keep pace

(a)

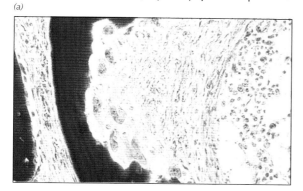

(b)

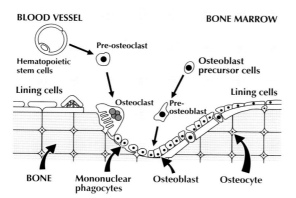

STRONG BONES – AN EVOLUTIONARY PREROGATIVE?

Why should the body expend so much energy and raw materials on constantly remodelling adult bone? The necessity for fractures to be repaired with new bone of full strength, rather than the fibrous scar tissue typical of healing elsewhere in the body, could be one reason. But bone's capacity for self-repair may have evolved more as a by-product of a greater evolutionary necessity: reproduction. Suppose that bone ceased to be continuously remodelled once it was fully grown, and deteriorated slowly in quality while the muscles and other soft tissues continued to be regularly renewed, as indeed they are, all through life. Long-lived animals like man, wholly dependent on an elaborate bone structure, would then be in their skeletal prime only very briefly, right at the outset of their reproductive lives. Natural selection seems to have evolved a sounder strategy for propagating the species.

Bone and muscle are notable among human tissues for peaking in mass during the most reproductive period, 10–15 years after puberty and about 10 years after growth in height has ceased. The self-regenerative capacity which makes this possible in bone seems most unlikely to be a chance biological leftover from primitive ancestors, more of whose tissues may well have been able to regenerate themselves, as those of reptiles still can today. Bone must have won its right to life-long regeneration in the hard school of natural selection, through parents with sound skeletons being better able to breed and rear offspring. It may even have been vital to human evolution, in a way that healing of occasional fractures could never have been.

This is not mere idle speculation. It serves to highlight the fact that fertility and strong bones take off together in adolescence, and it may help to explain the timetable of bone loss in postmenopausal women and the elderly. Can it really be coincidence that the gradual loss of bone among women in their thirties and forties roughly parallels their slowly declining fertility, and then accelerates suddenly when they become infertile at the time of the menopause? Surely it cannot be chance that bone loss in men, who normally remain fertile into old age, is deferred for at least another 20 years before senile osteoporosis develops? Whatever the precise reasons, the pattern is unmistakeable. Bone develops its strength in parallel with fertility and gets caught up in a running battle with osteoporosis only when the needs of reproduction have been served.

NEW BONES FOR OLD

The lifelong struggle to build up strong bone and then retain as much as possible need not be lost but can never be conclusively won. It is constantly waged in normal and osteoporotic bone by the small armies of specialized cells responsible for its modelling and remodelling: *osteoclasts*, which break down old bone, and *osteoblasts*, which replace it by building up new bone. They are both active at countless remodelling sites scattered throughout the skeleton, painstakingly renovating their way through the bones, and eventually starting all over again. A third type of bone cell, the *osteocyte*, is more of a staid housekeeper responsible for day-to-day maintenance of surrounding bone.

It takes no direct part in the remodelling process but appears to issue chemical instructions for its timing and location, a process known as *activation*.

(a)

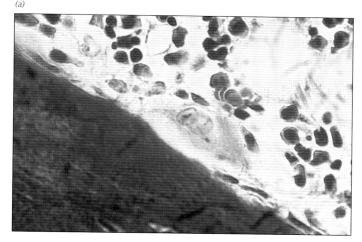

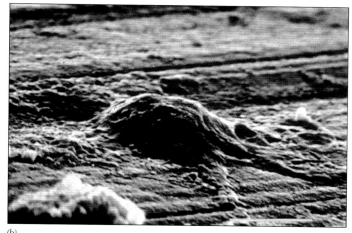

(b)

Figure 4
An osteoclast clearing a remodelling site by resorption of trabecular bone from one of its internal surfaces (a). Osteoclasts are multinucleated compound cells equipped for this purpose with a 'ruffled border' – the pale zone between cell and mineralized bone (stained blue). This contains cytoplasmic extensions, revealed by scanning electron microscopy (b), for resorbing the bone surface

As specialized demolition workers, the osteoclasts (*Figure 4*) are dedicated to clearance of remodelling sites, including those adjacent to fractures, for the osteoblasts to start building work on. Each osteoclast is a large compound cell with multiple nuclei, equipped with numerous processes to gnaw away at internal bone surfaces. Their brutish appearance (*see Figure 4*), and the speed with which they work might suggest that osteoclasts would perform the simple task of breaking down bone without much refinement. In reality they work with great precision, to a strict timetable, leaving no debris, and without disturbing neighboring bone. Once activated, these model demolition workers break down the hydroxyapatite and osteoid into their soluble constituents, which are then carried away by the bloodstream. Hence the description of their task as *resorption* of bone. It is so swiftly and subtly done, each remodelling site being cleared within a month, that even the osteoporotic victims of excessive bone resorption remain wholly unaware of the silent thieves stealing away their bones. The process of resorption produces no symptoms or signs whatever. And the surplus calcium released into the blood before being excreted in the urine does not provide clear evidence of bone loss, because it forms only a relatively small part of the normal blood levels and high daily turnover. Reliable tests for specific breakdown products of bone's collagen matrix (detailed in Chapter 5) have been evolved in recent years, however, and are now beginning to be used for investigating the rate of bone resorption.

The osteoblasts (*Figure 5*) are smaller cells, painstakingly working in construction teams responsible for building up new bone. This they do in two overlapping stages, over a total period of about 3–6 months, starting with formation of the organic bone matrix or osteoid. Its type-I collagen and other constituents are all synthesized and secreted by the osteoblasts themselves from raw materials delivered by the bloodstream. Amino acids provide ready-made building blocks for collagen and other matrix proteins, while calcium phosphate and the other mineral salts form hydroxyapatite. In fashioning the matrix for each part of every bone, the osteoblasts are responsible for building and maintaining the characteristic structure of the entire skeleton. As teams of osteoblasts each work on their own small sections of the osteoid matrix, these busy construction workers also produce a specific enzyme, bone alkaline phosphatase, which promotes its mineralization. The enzyme then passes into the bloodstream, where its concentration provides a test for gauging the rate of new bone formation in the body as a whole.

IMBALANCED RENEWAL – THE 'CAUSE' OF OSTEOPOROSIS

The work of the osteoclasts and osteoblasts never ends. Whenever work on one remodelling site is complete, it starts up in another. If this remodelling did not continue actively throughout life, adult bone would be unable to adapt to changing circumstances, and there would be no experienced and suitably specialized workforce on hand to repair fractures promptly with strong new bone. In bone weakened by osteoporosis, the osteoclasts and osteoblasts each continue to

perform their closely coordinated renewal work much as usual. However, the chemical mediators which enable new bone formation to be synchronized with resorption fail to keep these processes quantitatively in step with one another. Whether the deficit is small or large, it is hard to detect because it represents only a small fraction of the bone turnover constantly taking place in both normal and osteoporotic bone. Such deficits always arise from rates of resorption with which bone formation fails to keep pace, leaving remodelling sites incompletely filled with new bone. Osteoporosis may, therefore, arise from enhanced resorption, diminished formation, or both combined. But why should the body allow this imbalance to persist, even when it is progressively depleting the bones?

Local feedback control between the small groups of osteoclasts and osteoblasts beavering away at countless, widely-scattered remodelling sites could hardly be expected to perceive the overall picture, much less remedy any slight imbalance in the body as a whole. That calls for centralized control mechanisms. All aspects of bone growth and metabolism are, therefore, regulated by the interplay of systemic hormones acting on osteo-

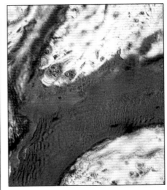

Figure 5
Trabecular bone is constantly remodelled on its numerous internal surfaces (*see Figure 10*). Large osteoclasts are resorbing one side of this trabecula, while smaller osteoblasts build new bone on the other, first forming collagen matrix which they then mineralize. Incomplete refilling of remodelling sites leads to bone loss and eventually to osteoporosis

Figure 6
Some of the many systemic and local factors which influence remodelling, acting directly or indirectly on osteoclasts and osteoblasts, which also exert feedback control over each other. The sex hormones, notably estradiol in women and testosterone in men, influence such mechanisms at several levels, keeping resorption and new bone formation in balance

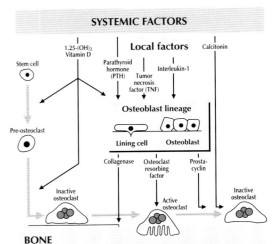

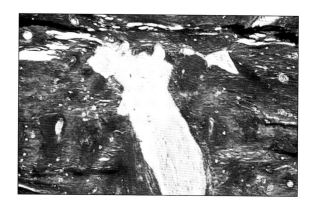

Figure 7
Cortical bone is remodelled at a lower rate, by tunnelling a 'cone' into its compact structure, because it lacks internal surfaces. Osteoclasts are continuing to cut out the upper part of this cone, while the lower part is already lined by osteoblasts refilling it with collagen matrix, which they will then mineralize to form a new osteon (*see Figure 9*)

Figure 8
Osteocytes like this one are specialized osteoblasts, permanently embedded in new bone as it is laid down. They appear to activate remodelling as well as regulating the metabolism and mineral content of all bone. Their numerous cytoplasmic tentacles, which run through fine tubular canaliculi in the bone, form an extensive network to communicate with other osteocytes. Even finer microcanaliculi radiate into surrounding bone, presumably to sense and respond to changes in structure or stresses

clasts and osteoblasts at remodelling sites throughout the skeleton (*Figure 6*). Several of them are now exploited, directly or indirectly, in the prevention and treatment of osteoporosis, as described in Chapter 6. The complex interplay of systemic factors responsible for regulating bone maintenance is not fully understood. Its detailed consideration lies outside the scope of this book – which is more concerned with their collective failure to maintain the status quo in adult bone. They very nearly succeed in doing so. Osteoporotic bone loss never represents more than marginal failure of the body's feedback systems to keep remodelling in balance

under adverse conditions. Yet these systems are plainly unable to control, or compensate sufficiently for, minor bone loss or the three most potent causes of osteoporosis: estrogen or testosterone deficiency, aging, and that twentieth century addition, corticosteroid therapy.

By their very nature, osteoclasts and osteoblasts perform specialized remodelling functions on the internal bone surfaces to which they are assigned (*Figures 5* and *7*), in much the same way as miners work their way along an underground coal face. Although their activities cause bone loss when they get out of phase, the cells can hardly be held responsible. They cannot perceive the overall results of their labors. The third type of bone cell, the housekeeping osteocyte, is much better situated to do that. Apparently responsible for day-to-day metabolism in the local bone matrix and for regulating its mineral content, the osteocytes form a three-dimensional network deeply buried within the matrix itself (*Figure 8*). Each keeps in constant touch with all its neighbors, thinly scattered throughout the bone, by means of slender cell processes. These must be responsible for coordinating osteocyte functions at local level, including activation of remodelling, but it is uncertain what part they may play in normal feedback control of the bone mass or its failure in osteoporosis.

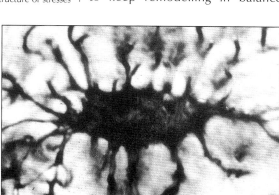

CORTICAL AND TRABECULAR BONE

Everything that has been said about the mineral, protein and cellular composition of bone applies to both its cortical and trabecular forms, despite their radical differences in structure. While cortical bone appears almost ivory-like in its solidity, it is far from inert, though it does have a less active metabolism, with fewer remodelling sites and a lower turnover than the more open-structured trabecular bone. The closely packed basic units of cortical bone known as *osteons* consist of concentric layers of bony lamellae around a central canal, which carries the blood supply (*Figure 9*). The sheer solidity of cortical bone means that it makes up a quite disproportionate 80% of the body's bone by weight, though occupying less than 50% of its total volume. Natural selection has, therefore, used its massive strength sparingly, where the need for it is compelling and unlikely to change much, mainly to withstand the leverage of powerful limb muscles on long bones and to carry the body's weight.

Trabecular bone looks more like a sponge (always enclosed in a hard outer crust of cortical bone), made up of a three-dimensional lattice-work of intersecting curved plates and tubes known as *trabeculae*, literally 'little beams' (*Figure 10*). These form intricate patterns of widely differing and often strikingly stylish design. All are genetically preprogrammed to combine maximum strength with relative lightness, not

just in a general way but so as to withstand the particular forces to which each part of a bone is normally subjected (*Figure 11*). Initially, the internal structure of trabecular bone thus develops to match its expected function. As it grows, and throughout adult life, it can also adapt, within limits, by responding to the stresses to which it is actually exposed – an observation embodied in Wolff's law. This states that a bone, normal or abnormal, develops the structure most suited to resist the forces acting upon it. Local feedback mechanisms are responsible for this. Mechanical stresses, probably mediated via the osteocytes, stimulate the remodelling process to form additional new

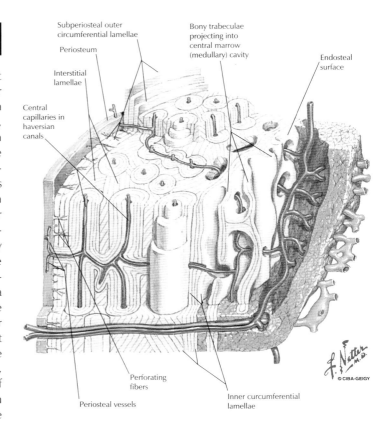

Figure 9
Cortical (or compact) bone from the shaft of a long bone, showing the densely packed cylindrical osteons which form most of its substance. Each is built up from concentric layers, resembling tree rings in their laminar structure and strength, but obtaining their blood supply from central capillaries (not external bark or periosteum). Bony lamellae pack the spaces between cylinders, giving greater rigidity

bone where it is needed most, just as an athlete's muscles build up in response to training. Trabecular bone is more responsive than cortical, a fact which also makes the already lightweight trabeculae more susceptible to bone loss under adverse conditions.

All long bones and most others contain both trabecular and cortical bone, judiciously arranged to serve their different functions by balancing the rival demands of strength, lightness and suitability for purpose. Thus the pipe-like shafts of the long bones consist almost exclusively of cortical bone, for its greater strength, whereas far lighter trabecular bone

fills out the expansions at each end and thus provides a slightly resilient base for joint surfaces, serving to minimize wear and tear (see *Figure 11a*). Trabecular bone is also to be found wherever a lightweight honeycomb provides a sufficiently robust structure for moderate weight-bearing – in the bodies of the vertebrae and parts of the pelvis, for example, or in the non-weight-bearing bone (*Figure 11b*) of the ilium or the scapula. Where lightness is of paramount importance, it even gives way to air-containing sinuses with thin bony walls, as in the human skull and the long bones of birds. Evolution is a cunning, experienced and flexible architect, not profligate with materials or undue weight, whose refined designs are not just constantly renovated but modified in the light of changing circumstances. This is both the source of bone's strength and of its weakness in osteoporosis.

If a particular bone proves to be unnecessarily strong for the limited demands to which it is exposed, its structure will adapt, also in accordance with Wolff's law, by remodelling itself to dispose gradually of the surplus. This is true both locally, of bone in an immobilized limb, for example, and of the skeleton as a whole when it is unstressed by weightbearing or exercise. The responsiveness of all bone, and of its trabecular form in particular, to a vast range of outside influences, for better or worse, is a striking feature of its development throughout childhood and adolescence.

Figure 10
Trabecular (or cancellous) bone, which typically forms the ends of long bones and the bodies of the vertebrae, has an open structure filled, like the hollow shafts of the long bones, with bone marrow. Compared with cortical bone, it has a higher blood supply with far more active metabolism and remodelling (lower part of diagram), which make it more susceptible to bone loss

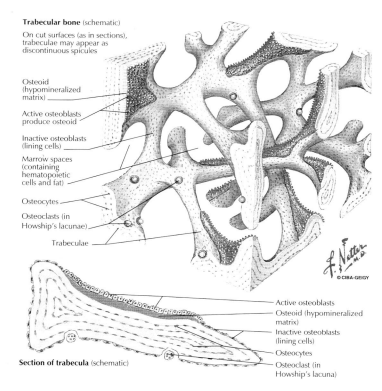

Trabecular bone (schematic)

On cut surfaces (as in sections), trabeculae may appear as discontinuous spicules

Osteoid (hypomineralized matrix)

Active osteoblasts produce osteoid

Inactive osteoblasts (lining cells)

Marrow spaces (containing hematopoietic cells and fat)

Osteocytes

Osteoclasts (in Howship's lacunae)

Trabeculae

Active osteoblasts
Osteoid (hypomineralized matrix)
Inactive osteoblasts (lining cells)
Osteocytes
Osteoclast (in Howship's lacuna)

Section of trabecula (schematic)

BONE FORMATION: GENETIC AND ENVIRONMENTAL INFLUENCES

Like every other tissue in the human body, bone grows in accordance with a precise program of genetic instructions, contained in and implemented by its constituent cells. From an early stage of fetal development, when the bones are first laid down as a sparingly mineralized collagen matrix, they are already exposed to hormones and other outside influences, from the baby's own body, from the mother's, and from her external environment. At the best, bone development will proceed apace, as it normally does, supplied with its essential needs. But we cannot take it for granted that everything is always for the best, even in that most protected of human environments, the pregnant uterus.

The more obvious defects of fetal bone development, such as the inherited form of brittle bone disease known as osteogenesis imperfecta, and the stunting of limb growth by thalidomide, are now clearly attributable to genetic and environmental causes, respectively. It is harder to be sure whether less devastating influences of either sort may predispose to later osteoporosis by impairing bone development less severely. The fragile bones of osteogenesis imperfecta break easily because of faults in one or more of the genes that code for their collagen matrix. Children with collagen defects not too severe to be compatible with survival have brittle bones highly susceptible to fracture. Minor genetic defects of collagen have not so far been established as predisposing causes of osteoporosis, but failure to synthesize sufficient collagen or minor abnormalities in its structure could lower the peak bone mass attainable in early adult life, which is known to be genetically influenced. Or genetic defects could conceivably produce matrix of lower durability, prone to premature deterioration and thus bone loss.

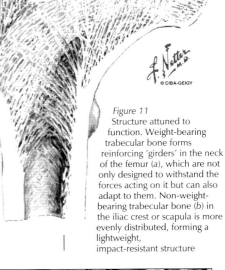

(a)

Figure 11
Structure attuned to function. Weight-bearing trabecular bone forms reinforcing 'girders' in the neck of the femur (a), which are not only designed to withstand the forces acting on it but can also adapt to them. Non-weight-bearing trabecular bone (b) in the iliac crest or scapula is more evenly distributed, forming a lightweight, impact-resistant structure

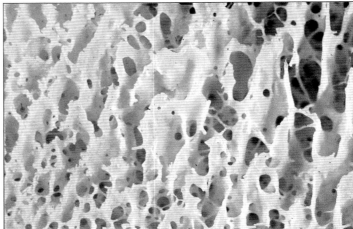

(b)

Early environmental factors more commonplace and much less damaging than thalidomide could also affect bone development before birth, with possible long-term ill effects. Cigarette smoking in pregnancy, for example, is known to inhibit cell division, and thus restrict fetal growth, reducing the average birth weight by about 225 g (8 oz). That the developing bones share in this generalized inhibitory effect on growth is clearly shown by a corresponding reduction in the length of babies born to smokers. Subsequent growth appears to be unaffected and there is no direct evidence at present linking predisposition to osteoporosis in later life with smoking in pregnancy. But anything that restricts normal development might impair the quality as well as reducing the quantity of bone collagen, thus lowering the peak bone mass and/or predisposing to bone loss later in life. We are only just beginning to understand how often the apparently negligible adversities of pregnancy can be visited on the future adult, in the form of schizophrenia, hypertension, and coronary heart disease, for instance. The bones may well be susceptible to such delayed ill effects.

BONE GROWTH: A PROPHYLACTIC OPPORTUNITY

Prevention of osteoporosis may be best regarded as a lifelong endeavor, starting before birth. It is never too early to start building up a strong skeleton. The emphasis should be on early prevention in girls, because they will reach a peak bone mass which is 25% lower, on average, than that in men. What women need is precisely the opposite: a larger skeletal reserve than men, to meet the greater future demands on it, particularly after the menopause. It is impossible to say why women should be doubly discriminated

against by having lower reserves of bone subject to earlier and much greater calls upon them. At first sight, genetically determined sex differences may appear to be responsible for both, but we cannot be sure that women are constitutionally condemned to bones so much lower in density. Given the opportunity, they might conceivably aspire to bone density closer to the present average in men, which may not be optimal either. That is a question for the future. The present reality is that women do have a considerably lower bone mass than men, and that they lose more of it earlier. Prevention of osteoporosis in later life calls for an unusually long perspective.

Genetic influences apart, the unborn child will normally receive adequate raw materials for building bone, notably amino acids, calcium, phosphate and vitamin D, via the placenta. If the mother's diet should be deficient in any of these essentials, the developing fetus tends to have priority, at her expense. At the same time, pregnancy normally protects the mother from bone loss because her estrogen levels are high. But plentiful pregnancy hormones, to which the developing fetus is also fully exposed, are no substitute for dietary deficiencies; they can only ensure that the available building materials are well absorbed and put to good use. It is, therefore, vital that pregnant women eat a good mixed diet, preferably with extra milk or calcium and vitamin D supplements. That the baby is exposed to maternal hormones including estrogens, as well as the interplay of its own growth, parathyroid and other hormones, all through pregnancy may well contribute to the normal development of its tissues in general and its bones in particular, provided that it receives all necessary nutrients for the purpose.

THE NEEDS OF GROWING BONES

A healthy child of either sex, who grows normally, consistently eats a good mixed diet containing adequate protein, minerals and vitamins, takes plenty of exercise, and matures sexually by the mid-teens, should attain a satisfactory, though not necessarily optimal, peak bone mass without any specific prophylactic measures. But not all children are healthy or grow up in such ideal circumstances, and girls will always be at higher risk even if they do. Failure to meet any of the optimal conditions for bone growth from infancy onwards may increase their risk of developing osteoporosis later in life, by imperceptibly reducing the bone they bank during childhood and adolescence.

A newborn baby's bones consist of relatively more osteoid matrix and less mineral than those of adults. At birth, the human skeleton contains only about 25 g (under an ounce) of calcium altogether, amounting to a little less than 1% of the average baby's birth weight. The proportion of the body weight represented by bone calcium roughly doubles during growth, approach-

ing 2% in an adult male. His skeleton would then contain an average of about 1200 g (over 2.5 lbs) of calcium. The actual bones weigh far more than this, of course, but it is clear that children's bones have a good deal of catching up to do, if their bone mineral is to rise at double their rate of growth. Given adequate supplies of calcium and vitamin D, they normally make a very good start, growing faster and increasing the body calcium more rapidly during the first 6 months, in proportion to body weight, than in any subsequent phase of growth. Normal breast or bottle feeding, sufficient to satisfy the baby, should provide more than the substantial supply of calcium required. Babies are genetically programmed to absorb it unusually well, aided by factors in milk which promote calcium absorption.

Appreciable levels of estradiol and other estrogens are always present in both human and cow's milk, with more progesterone in the latter, because a quarter or more of the cows in the herd from which milk is pooled will usually be in calf again. The large amount of calcium in milk and its ready availability, coupled with the presence of these (and possibly other) factors aiding its absorption, are probably the main reasons why more calcium is absorbed from milk and certain milk products than from green vegetables or other foods (Table 1). All ruminant animals are equipped with special digestive systems which not only extract calcium salts efficiently from grass and clover but also

Table 1 Calcium content of some of the best dietary sources (round figures in mg/100 g). The daily intake needs to exceed 1000 mg in young adults to compensate for normal excretion. The additional demands created by growth in adolescence and by accelerated rates of bone loss in the postmenopausal, elderly and others prone to osteoporosis require a higher daily intake, perhaps 1500 mg or more. Not all forms of calcium are well absorbed, vegetable sources not necessarily providing as much as dairy products or sardines with a similar calcium content

Dairy products		Fish (tinned, with bones)	
Milk	125	Sardines	350
Yoghurt	150	Tinned salmon	250
Cheddar cheese	750		
Dried milk	900	**Vegetables and nuts**	
Emmentaler	1150	Spinach, broccoli	100
		Kidney beans	100
Cereals		Kale	180
White bread*	85	Soya beans, dried	225
White flour*	265	Almonds	230
		Hazelnuts	250
Miscellaneous			
Milk chocolate	220		
Molasses	270		

Calcium is also present in meat, poultry, fresh fish, and other cereals, pulses and green vegetables, usually in lower concentrations. Taken together, these may represent a quarter or more of daily requirements

* Calcium enriched by law in UK

Figure 12
Cow's milk provides an ideal source of readily absorbed raw materials for growing bones. Like other ruminants, cows have digestive systems specially designed for extracting calcium and synthesizing first-class protein from large volumes of vegetable matter, which humans could neither tolerate nor put to such good use. Skimmed milk and some low-fat yoghurts contain even higher calcium and protein concentrations with little fat and fewer calories

convert this simple vegetarian diet into first-class protein. The human digestive system can do neither on anything like a comparable scale. Cow's milk and certain other dairy products, therefore, provide an unrivalled source of readily absorbed calcium, together with protein, fat, carbohydrate and vitamin D, first for the mother during pregnancy and breastfeeding and then for her growing child (*Figure 12*).

During the first year or so of life, when babies obtain most of their nourishment from breast or cow's milk, they normally tolerate it well. No substitute could be more easily digested or so readily provide calcium in sufficient quantities to satisfy the demands of growth. The estrogen levels in human and cow's milk expose the gut lining to concentrations sufficient to aid its absorption, especially in infancy, when milk is undiluted by much other food or drink. Once absorbed and distributed around a baby's body, the hormone concentration would be too low (unlike the period before birth) to have any appreciable effect on bone development or other body functions.

After the first birthday, however, some children become less able to digest milk because they lose the capacity to metabolize the milk sugar, lactose, which it always contains. All babies (and other young mammals) are genetically programmed to secrete an enzyme, lactase, specifically for this purpose, but its secretion wanes after the first year or so in most of the human race (and earlier in many other mammals). Only people of European extraction and others who presumably evolved alongside cattle retain the ability to synthesize lactase lifelong, though with some individual exceptions. About 5% of most European populations are thought to be lactase deficient, compared with over 90% of Chinese (which accords with the absence of milk and dairy products in traditional Chinese cuisine). Lactase deficien-

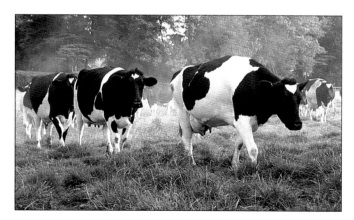

cy is not a complete bar to milk drinking, however. Those affected can usually tolerate a cupful or so a day, but that alone would not provide enough calcium for building strong bones. Inability to synthesize lactase, therefore, represents another genetic trait likely to diminish the peak bone mass and predispose to subsequent osteoporosis – particularly in orientals. Its ill effects could, of course, be overcome, if they were more widely recognized, by consuming adequate amounts of other calcium-rich foods or by taking a lactase preparation with milk.

Much of the high demand for body calcium in infancy is required for growth in the length and size of the bones, which will never be so fast again. Their mineralization rises only slightly, however. The bones therefore remain relatively bendy and resilient – thanks to their high osteoid content – during much of early childhood. Their flexibility probably enables them to grow more readily than if they were fully mineralized. It certainly means that children's bones often bend into relatively harmless 'greenstick' fractures if injured, instead of snapping. But, from infancy onwards, their relatively low mineral content combined with a high growth rate also makes them vulnerable to dietary deficiencies that might restrict normal development.

While full-blown rickets has become a rarity in the industrialized world, it does not necessarily follow that all children receive enough vitamin D, or calcium, for optimal growth and mineralization of their bones. The demand may outstrip available supplies after weaning onto more solid foods, especially if milk gives way to fruit juices or other drinks. Although vitamin D is normally synthesized in skin exposed to sunlight, there are only limited opportunities to expose much of a baby to the sun in temperate climates, especially for town-dwellers in the winter. Summer exposure may now be restricted for fear of skin cancer later in life. The best compromise must be a balanced diet containing plenty of calcium-rich foods with regular small supplements of cod-liver oil or other vitamin D preparations. This should not only prevent rickets but help to ensure that the growing skeleton develops its full genetic potential.

HIGH CALCIUM DEMAND

Calcium deficiency is the main dietary factor which may limit bone development, coming second only to inherited characteristics in its overall influence. For optimal growth in bone size and density, children and adolescents have to be continuously in positive calcium balance. In effect, the body has to absorb more calcium from food and drink than it continually loses via the urine, feces and, perhaps more surprisingly, the skin (in discarded scales and sweat). Because absorption is also far from complete, the diet always has to contain many times more calcium than the body needs to retain.

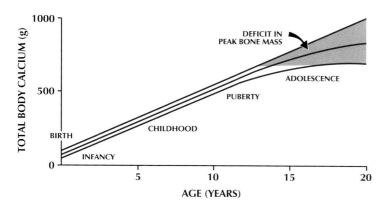

TOTAL BODY CALCIUM (g)

1000

500

0

BIRTH

INFANCY

CHILDHOOD

PUBERTY

ADOLESCENCE

DEFICIT IN
PEAK BONE MASS

5   10   15   20

AGE (YEARS)

Figure 13
'A girl of normal weight needs
to retain an average of 140 mg
extra calcium every single day
for 19 years, starting at birth.'
This high demand, which can
only be fully satisfied by a diet
containing 8 – 10 times as much
calcium is represented by the
straight line. In reality, demand
is higher in adolescence than in
childhood but less likely to be
met (shaded area) – which
diminishes the peak bone mass,
thus predisposing to
osteoporosis in later life

To achieve optimally developed
and mineralized bones by the end of
her teens (with a total body calcium
of about 1000 g), a girl of normal
weight needs to retain an average of
140 mg *extra* calcium every single
day for 19 years, starting at birth. In
practice, this high demand is not
evenly spread (*Figure 13*). It falls
towards the end of infancy and may
then be satisfied during childhood
by a well-balanced diet supplying at
least 1000 mg of calcium per day.
Many children do not reach that
total daily intake, and few exceed it
by much, even where hard water
makes an additional contribution.
The deficit should not be large,
however. Modest daily supplements
of milk and/or yoghurt, especially
desirable for girls growing up in soft
water areas, should ensure a positive
calcium balance throughout childhood.

That may no longer be true
when the demand for calcium rises
again with approaching adolescence. The growth spurt at puberty,
powered by the first impact of
testosterone in boys and of estradiol

in girls, nearly doubles the rate of
growth. This rises from around 5 cm
(about 2 inches) per year in late
childhood to 8.5 cm (well over 3
inches) in 12-year-old girls and to
9.5 cm (nearly 4 inches) in 14-year-
old boys, who typically undergo
puberty a year or two later. In both
sexes, but especially in girls, the
childhood period of bone growth is
now compressed by the progressively earlier occurrence of puberty in
industrialized societies. This tight
schedule makes it all the more
important that early bone development should be unimpeded. It is not
certain that any deficit which may
develop as a result of a foreshortened childhood can be made up
from puberty onwards – though it
probably could be with sufficiently
high calcium intake.

About 45% of the entire adult
bone mass should normally be
formed during adolescence, which
creates a formidable demand for
calcium that may not always be
satisfied. A corresponding increase
takes place in muscular strength,
particularly among adolescent boys,
in whom it normally doubles in
under 2 years. If fully exploited by
regular physical exertion, at sport or
work, the potential muscle power
stimulated by puberty further
strengthens the bones by stressing
the skeleton. But muscular and
skeletal development are not always
optimal today, with the decline in
active sport and manual labor
compounding the ill effects of calcium deficiency in many teenage
diets.

The demand for calcium peaks around the time of puberty and then remains high until growth is complete. Although the proportion of dietary calcium actually absorbed from the diet rises to its highest level in adolescence, there is also a substantial (though fortunately smaller) increase in calcium excretion, because more bone has to be resorbed for remodelling as growth accelerates. The daily requirement, therefore, rises above the childhood level, to about 1200 mg, which the calcium intake of the average teenager is most unlikely to reach. For adolescent girls, dietary calcium may fall further below the intake required for optimal bone development, which lies within a higher range of about 1200–1600 mg per day. But the milk drinking and more regular meals of childhood often give way to cola and erratic snacks at just this time. Calcium intake is, therefore, more likely to fall than rise to meet the greatly increased demand, with just one possible exception. The former craze for milk-shakes and the more recent taste for yoghurt, both most noticeable in teenage girls, may possibly owe something to an instinctive appetite for extra calcium at this critical stage of development. On balance, however, it is virtually certain that most teenage girls and many boys now lack sufficient calcium, and quite probably vitamin D as well, to build a skeleton as strong as their genes planned for them.

It might, of course, be claimed that today's teenagers are building bones strong enough for the relative-ly sedentary lives they are likely to lead, in an industrialized world no longer greatly dependent on human muscle power. But that argument is facile. It takes no account of the increase in postmenopausal and senile osteoporosis, which is not wholly attributable to greater longevity. It overlooks the unique opportunity to build up the bone mass in youth as a prophylactic measure. And it neglects the greater vulnerability of the female skeleton in later life.

ADVERSE INFLUENCES

Growth restriction

The bones of some children and teenagers are at additional risk from certain forms of long-term drug treatment, detailed in the next chapter. Corticosteroid therapy, which now poses the most common threat in this age group and is potentially the most serious, must be briefly considered here because it also affects growth. Given systemically for long periods, as these drugs quite often have to be in the treatment of chronic conditions (such as juvenile arthritis, severe asthma, certain skin conditions, and tumors), corticosteroids have three adverse effects on bone development. They restrict growth, hinder formation of new bone, and impair calcium absorption from the gut, all in proportion to dosage and duration of treatment. Corticosteroid ointments applied regularly to largish areas of skin can also be absorbed in sufficient quantities to have these effects. Even when inhaled regularly in low doses,

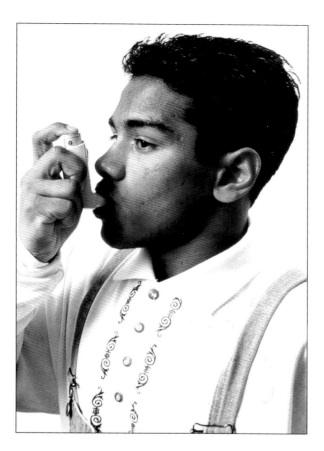

Figure 14
'Even when inhaled regularly in low doses, as preventive therapy for asthma, corticosteroids have been shown to reduce calcium absorption.' The adverse effect on bone mass is less serious than with systemic corticosteroid therapy but may be more insidious, being both unsuspected and unaccompanied by any warning signs

Limiting the peak bone mass

Compared with boys, girls typically have bones that are not only less strongly built, and stop growing sooner, but may be exposed to a wider range of adverse influences from early adolescence onwards. These commonly include lack of strenuous exercise to stress the bones, over-enthusiastic slimming, anorexia, and deficient diets (especially those containing no meat or dairy products, and therefore quite possibly deficient in protein as well as calcium and vitamin D). But by far the most important threat to bone development from the expected time of puberty is estradiol or testosterone deficiency. Delayed sexual maturation defers (or, in a few unfortunate teenagers who fail to mature sexually, precludes) both the adolescent growth spurt and the great strengthening of the bones that normally accompanies it. Once again, girls are at higher risk.

Amenorrhea and estrogen deficiency

Sometimes menstruation fails to start at about the normal age or does not become established in regular monthly cycles. Other adolescent girls start menstruating more or less normally only to become amenorrheic again for months or years at a time. Such menstrual irregularities almost invariably mean that ovulation is equally irregular. In the absence of ovulation, there will be no active ovarian follicle each month to secrete estradiol. Without adequate estradiol levels, a young

as preventive therapy for asthma, corticosteroids have been shown to reduce calcium absorption, apparently as a result of the small amounts that are swallowed acting locally on the gut lining (*Figure 14*). In adults, as the next chapter shows, long-term corticosteroid therapy is a potent cause of insidious bone loss and osteoporosis as such. While this can also occur in children and adolescents, the main effects in them are to restrain new bone formation and diminish its mineralization, thus limiting growth, and lowering the peak bone mass.

teenage girl's bones cannot develop fully; at the worst, bone loss may set in before the end of the teens.

Many otherwise healthy girls in their teens and twenties, and some with apparently unrelated problems, are now at risk in these ways, mainly because they are too thin for their height. If the proportion of body fat falls much below 18–20% of their total weight, the ovaries may either fail to become active at the normal age of puberty, or become inactive again later. As noted earlier, the teenage girls and young women at risk make a substantial but improbably assorted group, with little else in common, comprising athletes, gymnasts, ballet dancers, compulsive slimmers, anorexia and bulimia sufferers, heroin addicts, as well as emaciated victims of malnutrition or wasting diseases. Many of them are, of course, at additional risk from the ill effects of calcium lack and other dietary deficiencies on their bones. Even the intensive training and attention to diet among amenorrheic athletes and ballet dancers are insufficient to overcome the adverse effects of estrogen deficiency on the bones.

Infertility

From the early teens onwards, amenorrhea coupled with estradiol deficiency can also arise from endocrine or gynecological disorders associated with infertility, of which polycystic ovaries are the most frequent. Fortunately very rarely, the ovaries may need to be irradiated or removed in the teens or twenties,

producing an unusually early 'surgical' menopause. This necessitates estrogen replacement therapy, which is by no means always prescribed or taken regularly, to protect against bone loss. The same applies to the fortunately very rare instances of a premature menopause occurring spontaneously among young women in their late teens or twenties. In all such cases, concern about infertility understandably distracts attention from the risk of bone loss and the need for HRT.

Cigarette smoking

Finally, habitual cigarette smoking poses a risk to bone development in young women – and of bone loss in older ones – by partially depriving them of estradiol. Roughly in proportion to the number of cigarettes smoked, some of the estradiol normally produced is converted into an altered form which has no estrogenic activity itself and blocks estrogen receptors, thus partially inhibiting the activity of the remaining estradiol. No amenorrhea (or other warning sign) occurs in such cases to reveal that estradiol deficiency may be persistently weakening a female smoker's bones. Smoking has no effect on testosterone metabolism, so there is no corresponding risk in men.

Young men normally develop 30–50% stronger bones than girls during adolescence, and they are not exposed, then or later, to such a wide range of adverse influences. When youthful testosterone deficiency does occur, usually as a result of undescended testicles, it should nevertheless be taken seriously and corrected whenever possible. Both estradiol and testosterone play such active parts in the rapid bone development of adolescence, and its subsequent build-up to peak bone mass, that even marginal deficiency in the teens and twenties is bound to exert some adverse effect. Since individual hormone levels must be genetically determined, at least in part, this may well be yet another mechanism by which inherited characteristics influence the peak bone mass – and the long decline that follows.

Bibliographical notes

The growth, structure and remodelling of bone are described and illustrated by Dr Frank Netter in Vol. 8, Part 1 of the *Ciba Collection of Medical Illustrations* [Ciba-Geigy Corporation, Summit, New Jersey, 1987]. The Danish book *Knoglevaevets biologi* by Dr Leif Mosekilde [Ciba-Geigy A/S, Copenhagen, 1989] reviews bone structure and function with particular reference to osteoporosis. Gregory R. Mundy gives the most up-to-date and comprehensive account of *Bone Remodeling and its Disorders* [Martin Dunitz, London, 1995].

Evidence of the importance of calcium intake first came from a comparative study of fracture rates in hard and soft water areas [Matkovic V. (1979), Bone status and fracture rates in two regions of Yugoslavia, *Am. J. Clin. Nutr.*, **32**, 540–9], followed by detailed studies in the USA [Matkovic V. (1992), Calcium and peak bone mass, *J. Intern. Med.*, **231**, 151–60]. Milk is, however, a far more important source of calcium, especially in adolescence [Lindsay R. and Nieves J. (1994), Milk and bones; You are what you drink, *Br. Med. J.*, **308**, 930–1]. The whole field of 'Osteoporosis and Calcium' is concisely reviewed by L. Mosekilde (1992) introducing a minisymposium [*J. Intern. Med.*, **231**, 145–9], which includes: 'The scientific basis of recommended dietary allowances of calcium' by G. Schaafsma (1992) [*J. Intern. Med.*, **231**, 187–94], requirements at different ages, considered by R.P. Heaney (1992) [Calcium in the treatment and prevention of osteoporosis, *J. Intern. Med.*, **231**, 169–80], and a comparison of different dietary sources by P. Charles (1992) [Calcium absorption and calcium bioavailability, *J. Intern Med.*, **231**, 161–8]. Absorption is also covered by R.P. Heaney *et al.* (1990) [Absorbability of calcium sources: The limited role of solubility, *Calcif. Tissue Int.*, **46**, 300–4] who previously showed how uptake was improved by taking calcium with food [Heaney R.P. *et al.* (1989), Meal effects on calcium absorption, *Am. J. Clin. Nutr.*, **49**, 372–6]. More recently, T. Teegarden *et al.*

(1994) reported that 'Calcium supplementation increases bone density in adolescent girls' [*Nutr. Rev.*, **52**, 171–3], and E. Seeman *et al.* (1993) have considered 'Peak bone mass, a growing problem?' [*Int. J. Fertil. Menopausal Stud.*, **38 Suppl. 2**, 77–82].

Other determinants of bone mass at maturity have also been reviewed recently [Toss G. (1992), Effect of calcium intake vs. other life-style factors on bone mass, *J. Intern. Med.*, **231**, 181–6; Odell W.D. and Hunter H. (1993), Osteoporosis: Pathophysiology, Prevention, Diagnosis, and Treatment, *Disease-a-Month*, **XXXIX**, 804–7], and the peak attained in early adult life related to the fracture risk in older women [Hansen M.A. *et al.* (1991), Role of peak bone mass and bone loss in postmenopausal osteoporosis: 12-year study, *Br. Med. J.*, **303**, 961–4]. The value of exercise in promoting bone strength, as well as the risk of excessive activity causing amenorrhea, estradiol deficiency and consequent bone loss in young women, have been reviewed by R.L.Wolman (1994) [*ABC of Sports Medicine:* Osteoporosis and exercise, *Br. Med. J.*, **309**, 400–3]. Other studies have shown that adolescents need both adequate dietary calcium and physical exercise [e.g. Tylavsky F.A. *et al.* (1992), Are calcium intakes and physical activity patterns during adolescence related to radial bone mass of white college-age females? *Osteoporosis Int.*, **2**, 232–40]. The local effects of stress on particular bones are the subject of recent reports [Haapasalo H. *et al.* (1994), Long-term unilateral loading and bone mineral density and content in female squash players, *Calcif. Tissue Int.*, **54**, 249–55; Vuori I. *et al.* (1994). Effects of unilateral strength training and detraining on bone mineral density and content in young women: A study of mechanical loading and deloading on human bones, *Calcif. Tissue Int.*, **55**, 59–67].

Multiple factors appear to determine inherited predisposition to osteoporosis [Brandi M.L. *et al.* (1994), Editorial: Genetics of Osteoporosis, *Calcif. Tissue Int.*, **55**, 161–3; Pocock N.A. *et al.* (1987), Genetic determinants of bone mass in adults, *J. Clin. Invest.*, **80**, 706–10], though a single gene has been claimed to exert a major influence on bone density [Morrison N.A. *et al.* (1994), Prediction of bone density from vitamin D receptor alleles, *Nature*, **367**, 284–7; also comment by Mundy G.R. (1994), Boning up on genes, *Nature*, **367**, 216–17].

References to the adverse effects of smoking, excessive exercise, anorexia and of corticosteroid therapy follow Chapter 3.

Chapter 3:
Osteoporotic bone

A VICTIM OF CIRCUMSTANCE

When healthy bone becomes osteoporotic, it is primarily a victim of adverse circumstances, not diseased in itself or abnormal in its response to outside influences. It remains unchanged in outward appearance as its strength declines. Internally, trabecular and cortical bone each retain their distinctive characters, with little more than necessary adaptation to their progressive loss of structure. Even in advanced osteoporosis, the depleted bone consists of normally constituted collagen matrix, fully mineralized. There is simply too little of each. With the single exception of osteocyte depletion in old age, no inherent abnormality has been demonstrated in any of the components of normal bone which might account for it becoming osteoporotic. The osteoclasts and osteoblasts continue to perform their routine remodelling tasks – as the unwitting agents of bone loss, not its true causes. Busily resorbing old bone and replacing it with new, in accordance with outside instructions, they perpetrate the slight but persistent excess of bone resorption, which underlies all osteoporosis, because they have no choice. Technically guilty of stealing bone, they are hardly to blame for its loss.

The imbalance between resorption and bone formation does not arise from any known fault in the osteoclasts or osteoblasts themselves, from failure of the chemical communication between them, or from disordered responses to systemic hormones or other external influences. These invaluable cells not only continue to remodel osteoporotic bone but adapt to its loss of structure by maximizing the strength of what remains. Fractures in osteoporotic bone heal satisfactorily, because they continue to play their normal parts. The osteoclasts resorb the fractured bone ends and the osteoblasts immobilize them by forming roughcast callus in and around the break, before they collaborate to remodel it into trabecular or cortical bone, as appropriate to the site. With the development of specific forms of treatment for osteoporosis in recent years, it has become increasingly apparent that the osteoclasts and osteoblasts are also largely responsible for mediating their therapeutic effects in osteoporotic bone. The agents of bone loss can thus be recruited to its prevention and treatment.

In effect, the actions of osteoclasts and osteoblasts represent a final common pathway by which all outside influences affect bone remodelling, for better or worse, in osteoporotic as in normal bone.

They are as much victims of circumstance as the bone they deplete. The true causes of osteoporosis must therefore be sought outside these cells, most of them outside the bones affected, and some outside the body altogether. This chapter seeks to identify them. It examines the gradual decline from peak bone mass, always mediated by a slight but persistent imbalance in remodelling activity, the circumstances in which the net loss may accelerate, and the reasons why.

DECLINE COMES BEFORE A FALL

The long decline from peak bone mass normally begins by the early thirties, for reasons that cannot yet be fully explained. But it follows the familiar cyclical pattern of all life on earth. The sex hormones which spurred bone to its peak also appear to lie at the heart of its decline. The first fine rapture of the biological response to estradiol and testosterone that powered adolescence into early adulthood is already on the wane, perhaps for two reasons. By the early thirties, production of sex hormones appears to have passed its peak in both sexes, and the high physical and mental responsiveness of young tissues first exposed to their stimulating effects has begun to fade. Sexual activity, which is normally both stimulated by and stimulates secretion of the sex hormones, starts to lose some of its early fervor and may decline in frequency. Participation in sport and other activities becomes less energetic and peak performance falls. By the late twenties, the

muscles begin to lose some of their youthful bulk and power, and the body its youthful physique. The waist fills out and the skin starts to wrinkle, betraying the first signs of approaching middle age. Sooner than most people care to admit, it is downhill all the way, and not only for the bones.

The bone mass painstakingly built up during the first 25–30 years of life does not all peak at once in different bones, or at anything remotely like uniform levels throughout the body. There is not one peak bone mass but many, at various times in different parts of the skeleton, but typically occurring earlier in trabecular bone than cortical. Once the mass of a particular bone, or part of it, has peaked, it begins to decline within a few months or years (Figure 1). Starting slowly, again at various times in different parts of the skeleton, and running at diverse rates, this decline follows recognizable – though not always explicable – patterns.

Cortical bone may still be building up, when trabecular has already

Figure 1
The natural history of bone. After peaking by the age of about 30, the bone mass declines slowly at first, before accelerating at the menopause, in old age and under other adverse influences (represented by dotted lines). All such influences are cumulative, whether they diminish the peak bone mass in youth or cause bone loss later in life

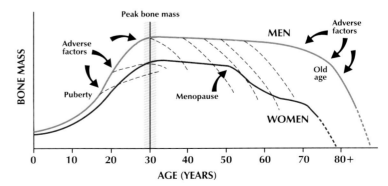

started to decline. The very fact that bone loss follows set patterns strongly suggests that local susceptibility must be genetically pre-programmed. Trabecular bone (with its open structure, greater blood supply, larger number of remodelling sites and higher turnover) is always more susceptible than cortical bone. In addition, rates of loss differ between bones of similar constitution and even between different parts of the same bone. On a larger scale, seemingly comparable individuals lose bone at widely differing rates, which are also influenced by their sex, age and ethnic origins. But genetic predisposition cannot be the sole cause of all this variability. Rates of bone loss must also be governed by the interplay of numerous factors – local, systemic and environmental – acting on the genetic substrate. It is the outcome of that complex interplay, as it evolves over time, which first determines the peak bone mass and then presides over its long decline, determining who will eventually become osteoporotic, how seriously, and when.

The progressive loss of bone that begins in the thirties would create few serious problems if it continued at its low initial rate, roughly matching the decline in muscular strength and activity with advancing age. That is what happens in most men, at least into their seventies, but not in women. For all of them, but for

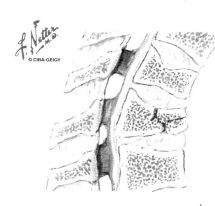

Figure 2
Compression fracture of vertebral body in a postmenopausal woman. The menopause is normally followed by rapid bone loss from the vertebral bodies, which may become fracture prone within 2 or 3 years. One or more may then collapse as a result of minimal trauma, often so slight as to be unnoticed

relatively few men, the natural history of bone has earlier hazards lying in wait. In more than one sense, the first years of gentle decline in bone mass come before a fall. Sooner or later, accelerated loss will be superimposed on the slow rate of decline – sooner in amenorrheic younger women and others at high risk, later in postmenopausal women, and much later still in the vast majority of men. The amount by which bone loss accelerates and its timing differ widely, however. Its rate can be low enough, even after the menopause, to pose no great risk of osteoporotic fractures over a normal lifespan. At the opposite extreme, the initial loss caused by estrogen deficiency can be so rapid that the most susceptible areas of trabecular bone lose 5–10% of their total mass in each of the first few postmenopausal years. Their strength can then fall below the notional 'fracture threshold' – the level at which bone breaks unduly easily – within 2 or 3 years. These are the circumstances in which recently postmenopausal women are liable to fracture their forearms or other limb bones in minor falls, or to sustain fractures of one or more vertebral bodies (*Figure 2*).

The high rates of accelerated bone loss responsible for such injuries usually settle down a few years after the menopause, apparently because the bones gradually acclimatize to estradiol deficiency. But accelerated bone loss cannot be relied upon to fall back to acceptably low levels unless its cause ceases or active countermeasures are taken. Few causes of bone loss are temporary or self-limiting. Some, like long-term corticosteroid therapy, do not abate at all, unless dosage is reduced or withdrawn. Whatever its cause, accelerated bone loss always calls for preventive therapy to reduce or even reverse that loss. Not many, even of those most at risk, yet receive it. How badly preventive therapy is needed will of course depend partly on the patient's age and sex but mainly on the two key factors which ultimately determine the severity of all osteoporosis: the peak bone mass and the cumulative effect of subsequent rates of loss. The various influences which can prevent the peak bone mass from attaining its full potential, especially in girls, were outlined in the last chapter. There are at least equally compelling reasons, most of them similar in nature, why bone loss should eventually accelerate, typically putting women's bones at greater risk than men's.

AMENORRHEA AND PREMENOPAUSAL BONE LOSS

There are several circumstances in which the slow decline from peak bone mass may accelerate within a few years. Many of them are peculiar to women of childbearing age. The commonest type of bone loss to which they are uniquely prone is premenopausal in its timing but postmenopausal in nature. Its unsuspecting victims are women in their thirties and forties who either already are or have become estradiol deficient, whatever the reason. They lose bone prematurely as a

result and may begin to develop Type I osteoporosis at any time during the 20–25 years which normally separate the attainment of peak bone mass from the menopause. For want of screening programs, this may not become apparent for many years, when their osteoporosis has resulted in fractures. Cause and effect are then too remote for the connection to be obvious. For this and other reasons, the potentially serious effect of hormone deficiency on the bones of younger women is still neglected. The condition even lacks a distinctive name. Here it will be described simply as *premenopausal bone loss*, to reflect both its timing and its nature.

The estradiol deficiency which underlies it can develop for the first time in adulthood, or it may simply be a continuation of the earlier deficiency which impaired the attainment of peak bone mass following puberty. Persistent amenorrhea (or very infrequent menstruation) is again the principal warning sign. It may still be caused by low body weight among adult athletes, joggers, dancers, anorectics and the others discussed earlier, though most of these 'occupational' factors become less common with age. Amenorrhea may also be associated with any endocrine or gynecological disorder which prevents the ovarian follicles from ovulating and secreting estradiol. Causes of this kind increase with age, as does the risk of a premature menopause occurring spontaneously or needing to be surgically induced.

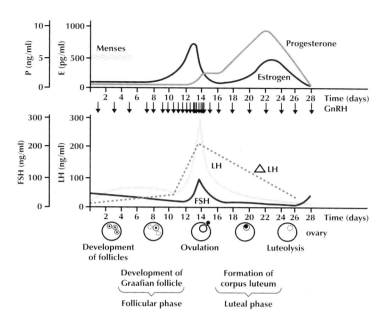

Figure 3
The normal ovarian cycle, showing the follicular or preovulatory phase when estradiol (E) secretion is predominant, followed by ovulation and the luteal or progestational phase in which progesterone (P) prepares the endometrium for implantation of the ovum or the onset of menstruation. Except in pregnancy, amenorrhea shows that the cycle is inoperative and the patient estrogen-deficient. Pulses of GnRH (gonadatropin releasing hormone) normally stimulate secretion of LH (luteinizing hormone) and FSH (follicle stimulating hormone), which act on the ovaries. Reproduced from Fink, G. (1979). *Br. Med. Bull.*, **35**, 155, with permission from Churchill Livingstone

Whatever its underlying cause, the estradiol deficiency associated with amenorrhea is the crucial factor. As a general rule, non-pregnant women of childbearing age who are not menstruating will not be ovulating regularly either and must therefore be both infertile and estrogen deficient – at least for the time being – whether they have flushes and other withdrawal symptoms or not. If their normal ovarian cycle cannot be restored (*Figure 3*), they need HRT, irrespective of age, to protect them from osteoporosis, to maintain their libido, to enhance mood, and to reduce the risk of premature cardiovascular disease. Otherwise they will be exposed to a high risk of accelerated bone loss, and of heart attacks, especially if predisposed by estradiol deficiency earlier in life, which also prevented them from attaining an adequate peak bone mass.

HORMONE REPLACEMENT THERAPY IN YOUNGER WOMEN

The case for estrogen replacement is overwhelming in younger women with persistent amenorrhea. They need normal estradiol levels more than postmenopausal women because they are at risk earlier and therefore more prone to prolonged bone loss and premature cardiovascular disease. Sadly, that need often goes unrecognized in practice. At present, only a minority of estrogen-deficient younger women receive appropriate treatment. Few of the minority who are given HRT (or an oral contraceptive) take it for a sufficient period to safeguard their bones or protect their blood vessels. Even when the necessity for HRT has been created by a surgical menopause, it may be prescribed for only a minority of patients, and then be regarded as short-term therapy to control the hot flushes and other immediate symptoms of estradiol withdrawal.

Young women who seek medical advice about persistent amenorrhea or complain of infertility, hot flushes, depression, loss of libido or other symptoms suggestive of estradiol deficiency may be no better treated. Their need for estrogen replacement may not be understood by patient or doctor, preoccupied, as they often are, by the question of infertility. Few amenorrheic younger women have their natural cycles restored. Not many of the remainder are prescribed HRT at all, and not many of them continue to take it for long enough to protect their bones and blood vessels. Persistent amenorrhea deserves to be taken much more seriously as a sign of estradiol deficiency, and, therefore, as a major risk factor for cardiovascular disease and osteoporosis in all women of childbearing age.

CONSERVATION OF THE OVARIES

There are just two common exceptions to this rule. A younger woman may be amenorrheic, without being estrogen deficient, following a simple hysterectomy at which only the uterus was removed, leaving functional ovaries *in situ*. This procedure obviously precludes menstruation but does not prevent ovulation or cause estrogen deficiency. If gynecologists conserved the ovaries whenever possible, there would then be less need for HRT before the normal age of menopause (which may or may not be revealed by the subsequent onset of hot flushes and other estrogen withdrawal symptoms).

The second exception, pregnancy, is far from estrogen deficient and typically tends to strengthen rather than weaken the mother's bones. Certain pregnant women on low-calcium diets are, nevertheless, likely to sacrifice part of their own hard-won bone mass to their babies during pregnancy and lactation, probably by a process of accelerated bone resorption liberating calcium to make up the deficit. This risk could be reduced or averted altogether by a high-calcium intake with vitamin D supplements, but antenatal care seldom includes such measures, or even considers the long-term well-being of the mother's – or baby's – bones.

OSTEOPOROSIS OF PREGNANCY

An unusual and as yet unexplained form of osteoporosis develops more acutely during or soon after pregnancy in a few women, who typically present with acute back pain and may be found to have vertebral-body fractures. The probable explanation is that osteoclastic activity becomes overstimulated to break down and resorb trabecular bone, presumably to mobilize bone calcium, in a mistaken attempt to compensate for low blood levels – and thus avoid depriving the unborn child. Whatever its precise cause, increased awareness that unusually acute osteoporosis can present as back pain during or soon after pregnancy should lead to earlier diagnosis, limit its ill effects and help to clarify its nature. Women known to have had osteo-

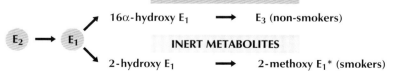

ACTIVE ESTROGENS

$E_2 \rightarrow E_1$

16α-hydroxy $E_1 \longrightarrow E_3$ (non-smokers)

INERT METABOLITES

2-hydroxy $E_1 \longrightarrow$ 2-methoxy E_1* (smokers)

* Receptor blocker (or other mechanism)

Figure 4
How smoking predisposes to osteoporosis in young women. Among non-smokers, estradiol (E_2) is normally metabolized to other active estrogens, including estrone (E_1) and estriol (E_3). In smokers, some estradiol is metabolized to an inert 2–methoxy derivative of estrone, which also blocks estradiol receptors, thus further inhibiting the action of the remaining hormone

porotic vertebral fractures in one pregnancy need to be monitored carefully during future pregnancies and followed up long-term, in case they are unusually prone to osteoporosis later in life.

SMOKING LOWERS ESTRADIOL LEVELS

Among other premenopausal causes of bone loss, cigarette smoking can contribute significantly to the risk of osteoporosis in normally menstruating women. It has three adverse effects on estrogen activity, two of them touched upon briefly in the last chapter. Smoking induces an enzyme change which results in substantial quantities of estradiol (proportional to the amount smoked) being converted into a metabolite, 2-methoxyestrone, which not only lacks estrogenic properties itself but also blocks estradiol receptors (*Figure 4*). The effect of this is both to reduce the concentration of estradiol circulating in the bloodstream and partially to block the action of what remains. In addition, the relative risk of early menopause is doubled in heavy smokers compared with women who have never smoked (*Figure 5*). This appears to result from absorption of (as yet unidentified) toxic components of tobacco smoke which reduce the number of viable follicles left in a woman's ovaries as she approaches the menopause. When there are only a few hundred left, both estradiol production and menstruation cease, and bone loss accelerates – a year or two prematurely.

The cumulative effect of heavy smoking on a middle-aged woman's skeleton is severe enough to have earned its own epithet – 'smoker's bones'. Smoking appears to have little toxic action on bone metabolism, however, since there is less evidence of bone loss being more severe in postmenopausal or male smokers. Just one note of caution needs to be added: the ill effects of heavy smoking on estradiol metabolism are not confined to the naturally produced hormone. Estradiol taken by postmenopausal women as HRT must be modified by smoking in the same way. Its effective concentration must, therefore, be reduced in smokers, limiting both its short-term efficacy in relieving menopausal symptoms and its long-term value in protecting the bones and cardiovascular system. This could be one of the reasons why HRT sometimes fails to curb postmenopausal bone loss.

Some forms of long-term drug therapy and/or exposure to pollution may also have direct toxic effects on the ovarian follicles – impairing estradiol production and/or advancing the menopause. Certain cytotoxic drugs and radiotherapy used to treat cancer and

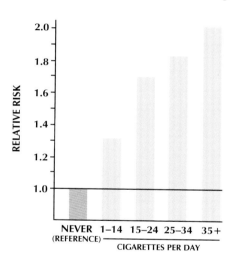

RELATIVE RISK

2.0
1.8
1.6
1.4
1.2
1.0

NEVER 1–14 15–24 25–34 35+
(REFERENCE)
CIGARETTES PER DAY

Figure 5
Smoking not only impairs estradiol activity, it also increases the relative risk of an early menopause. Estradiol secretion therefore ceases prematurely, advancing the onset of postmenopausal bone loss in women whose bone density will already have been lowered by years of smoking

leukemia obliterate the ovarian follicles, producing an immediate menopause with consequent estradiol deficiency. Although the resulting bone loss could be classed as secondary, it would be confined to women, result from estrogen deficiency, and therefore be postmenopausal in type.

SECONDARY OSTEOPOROSIS

All osteoporosis is secondary to internal or external factors, most of which have now been identified. However, the term 'secondary' (sometimes called Type III) osteoporosis is normally reserved for bone loss caused by factors other than estrogen deficiency and aging. Lack of stress on the bones, its simplest form, seldom amounts to more than a contributory cause, generally attributed to the decline in manual labor. Prolonged bedrest became a rarity as a form of treatment nearly 50 years ago, once chemotherapy had been developed for tuberculosis. But many disabled people are at risk today, the degree and distribution of their secondary bone loss always depending on the severity and duration of their disability and the parts of the body not exposed to muscular or gravitational stress. While the severe bone loss experienced by astronauts during long periods of weightlessness is hardly likely to become commonplace, barring the introduction of packaged space travel, it at least serves to remind us of the importance of weight-bearing, as well as muscular exertion, in maintaining strong bones. In the absence of either,

remodelling will always downgrade relevant parts of the skeleton for lighter duties.

Most secondary osteoporosis takes the very different form of bone loss caused by diseases or drugs (*Table 1*). These operate by a variety of mechanisms, alone or in combination, which ultimately enhance resorption of bone, diminish its formation, or adversely affect the absorption or excretion of calcium. Only a few of the drugs which cause secondary osteoporosis are potentially serious, most doing only limited harm on their own, even if continued long-term. Drug-induced osteoporosis might, therefore, be considered of secondary importance – as no more than a contributory factor adding to the severity of post-menopausal or senile bone loss – were it not for corticosteroids.

CORTICOSTEROID THERAPY – A POTENT CAUSE OF BONE LOSS

Corticosteroids are now so widely prescribed in industrialized countries, for as much as 15–20% of the adult population at one time or

Table 1 Causes of secondary osteoporosis, many of which act via familiar mechanisms: lack of estradiol or testosterone, corticosteroid excess, impaired calcium absorption, physical inactivity. All such causes are cumulative and can act only by reducing the bone mass attained in youth or accelerating its subsequent loss

LIFESTYLE

Inactivity (bed rest, weightlessness)
Smoking (women of childbearing age)
Alcoholism

DIETARY DISORDERS

Calcium/vitamin D deficiency
Malnutrition/malabsorption
Vitamin C deficiency (scurvy)
High protein intake (in elderly)
High phosphate intake

SEX–HORMONE DEFICIENCY

Premature or surgical menopause
Amenorrhea/polycystic ovaries
Testosterone deficiency in men

OTHER ENDOCRINE DISORDERS

Cushing's disease
Hypopituitarism
Thyrotoxicosis
Diabetes
Addison's disease
Acromegaly

BONE AND BONE MARROW DISEASES

Metastatic carcinoma
Leukemia, myeloma, lymphoma
Hemophilia, thalassemia

KIDNEY OR LIVER DISEASE

Renal failure/dialysis
Aluminum overload
Hepatic failure/cirrhosis

DRUG TREATMENT (LONG-TERM)

Corticosteroids
Antacids (aluminum-based)
Anticoagulant (heparin)
Immunosuppressants (e.g. methotrexate)
Anticonvulsants (phenobarbitone, phenytoin)

another, that they have become by far the commonest cause of secondary osteoporosis. They are also one of the most potent, high-dosage long-term therapy being capable of inducing annual losses of 10% or more of trabecular bone. In adults, systemic corticosteroids both impair calcium absorption from the gut and inhibit new bone formation, the main difference from their effects in childhood and adolescence being that there is no longer any growth to be inhibited.

Bone loss begins within days of starting systemic corticosteroid treatment, as resorption is no longer counterbalanced by new bone formation. Its severity depends on the dosage and duration of therapy. High doses taken for more than a few weeks or moderate doses for months or years are the main risks capable of causing profound osteoporosis even in the absence of other adverse factors. The already high risk in young adults rises further with age, as more people develop conditions calling for corticosteroid therapy and become more prone to bone loss for other reasons. These losses will inevitably be cumulative, and almost as inevitably be compounded in due course by postmenopausal and/or senile osteoporosis.

Prescribers of long-term corticosteroid therapy seldom take its potentially devastating effects on the bones fully into account. Well-meaning attempts are normally made to keep the dosage to a minimum and/or limit the duration of therapy, but that is usually all.

Probably the fact that corticosteroids were introduced into clinical medicine over 30 years before densitometry and other reliable diagnostic tests became available accounts for the establishment of this unsatisfactory practice. Its continuance today is harder to justify. Densitometry is still not performed routinely to check the bone mineral content of patients taking long-term corticosteroids, much less repeated at intervals to establish the rate of bone loss. Without such factual information as a guide, the prescriber can only guess what is happening to the patient's bones and hope for the best. The usual practice of keeping total dosage to a minimum may be better than nothing, but it ignores the fact that there is no therapeutically effective dosage of systemic corticosteroids low enough to leave the bones entirely unscathed.

Local osteoporosis

Secondary osteoporosis is sometimes a purely local phenomenon, confined to particular bones or parts of them. It may be caused by such local factors as immobilization of a limb or rheumatoid arthritis in a neighboring joint. The local bone loss does not affect the rest of the skeleton, and can be controlled, so far as may be possible, by correcting the local cause. It need not concern us further here, except as a reminder that bone loss is always determined by local as well as systemic influences, just as exercise strengthens the muscles and bones subjected to stress, rather than the entire musculature and skeleton. Local factors, determined genetically as well as by exertion and other environmental influences, must also be responsible for the local patterns of bone loss that are highly characteristic of post-menopausal and senile osteoporosis.

PATTERNS OF BONE LOSS – AND ADAPTIVE CHANGES

The timings and rates of loss from different bones, even from different parts of the same bone, are much more diverse than generalized causes like estradiol deficiency, cortico-steroid therapy or old age can adequately explain. Local rather than systemic factors must clearly contribute to the wide, but remarkably consistent, local variations observed in the timing of onset and the severity of osteoporosis.

Trabecular bone loss

The most striking early change occurs in women, starting many years before the menopause. Trabecular bone is lost initially from the neck of the femur, particularly from the area known as Ward's triangle (*Figure 6*), starting at a rate of about 0.5% each year. This gradually rises as estradiol levels decline, so that, by the time of the menopause, that part of the neck of the femur may have lost as much as 30% of its mineral content. That is more than other weight-bearing parts of the skeleton which have been investigated, quite probably more than any other bone at this comparatively early stage, despite the crucial importance of the femoral neck and its constant expo-

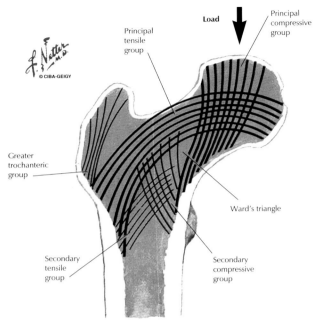

Trabecular groups conform to lines of stress in weight bearting

sure to the stresses of weight-bearing and everyday activities. The early onset and severity of this local bone loss is also at odds with the long-deferred risk of femoral neck fracture, which does not rise sharply until the late seventies. The delay of 25 years or more is hard to explain in terms of bone loss alone. More probable explanations are the many factors which increase the risk of old people falling heavily, since these rise roughly in parallel with hip fractures, plus the likelihood that bone quality may deteriorate in old age, out of proportion to its loss.

Trabecular bone in the trochanteric region of the femur (despite being close to the areas of severe premenopausal bone loss) and in the vertebral bodies does not

Figure 6
Load-bearing in the head, neck and upper shaft of the femur. The trabeculae transfer the body weight to cortical bone in the shaft – particularly via the compressive group, acting as a supporting pillar, and the tensile group which resemble an arch or prestressed lintel. The critical area of Ward's triangle, from which bone starts to be lost before the menopause, lies between them

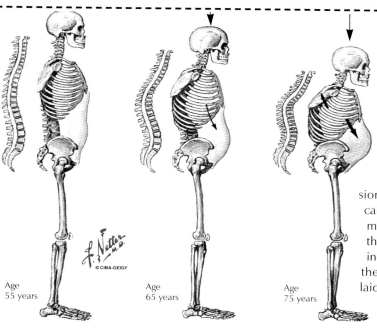

Age
55 years

Age
65 years

Age
75 years

Figure 7
Progressive spinal deformity and loss of height in a postmenopausal woman. Once mid-thoracic kyphosis has set in, further bone loss conspires with adverse spinal mechanics to increase the resulting deformity (see *Figure 22* in Chapter 6). The diaphragm and viscera are then pushed further downwards and forwards, distending the abdomen and eventually bringing the lower ribs into (painful) contact with the iliac crest

start to lose density rapidly much before the menopause. Thereafter the loss becomes very rapid in some women, reaching as much as 10% from the central region of the vertebral bodies in each of the first two postmenopausal years. This is among the highest annual rates recorded for any bone. Though the early susceptibility of the vertebral bodies is inexplicable at present, it does accord with the predominance of vertebral-body fractures soon after the menopause. The resulting deformity often continues to deteriorate in old age (*Figure 7*).

Changes in cortical bone

Cortical bone (usually studied in the shaft of the radius, for its technical convenience) behaves very differently. Its density goes on increasing into the thirties, beyond the average time of peak bone mass, suffers no appreciable loss before the menopause, and declines relatively slowly (by no more than 2–3% per annum) thereafter. In these respects, it appears to follow the same pattern of cortical loss seen in the shafts of other long bones. The characteristic thinning of cortical bone, which is its main concession to bone loss, whatever the cause, takes place from within. The marrow cavity in the shafts of all the long bones gradually enlarges, increasing the internal diameter. At the same time, some new bone is laid down externally, enlarging the external diameter, though not to the same extent. This helps to compensate for the overall thinning of the cortex (*Figure 8*), by making optimal use of the remaining bone, in accordance with Wolff's law and sound engineering principles. It also shows that osteoporotic cortex retains its capacity to respond adaptively to stress, so as to obtain maximal strength from limited raw materials.

Trabecular adaptation

The more fundamental osteoporotic changes that afflict trabecular bone before and after the menopause are also accompanied by adaptive attempts to put its diminishing structure to optimal use and thus maintain its mechanical strength for as long as possible. These adaptive changes can be clearly seen in the vertebral bodies. As the three-dimensional trabecular framework becomes thinned, and loses the stabilizing effect of some of its cross-members when they rupture, the remaining vertical components gradually thicken to form slender arches known as arcades (*Figure 9*). In their marriage of engineering principles with elegance, some of these bear a striking resemblance to the soaring arches of gothic cathedrals, which were of course specifically designed to carry massive weight on a relatively light open-work structure (typically consisting of limestone, which resembles hydroxyapatite in its structural properties). Adaptation of this kind must prevent many vertebral fractures, although it represents no more than a holding operation in the course of a losing battle. Eventually, the osteoporotic bone can adapt no further and becomes increasingly vulnerable to fracture if bone loss continues.

POSTMENOPAUSAL (TYPE I) OSTEOPOROSIS

Amenorrhea is associated with estradiol deficiency and thus with osteoporosis, before or after the menopause, because absence of menstruation generally signifies lack of ovulation. It is the process of ovulation, by which a follicle in one or other ovary normally produces an ovum each month, which is also responsible for estradiol production, not the ovaries themselves (*see Figure 3*). But there is a crucial difference between amenorrhea in a premenopausal woman, which is potentially reversible, and the permanence of the menopause, whenever it occurs. When ovulation, and therefore estradiol produc-

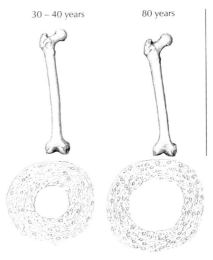

30 – 40 years   80 years

Figure 8
Adaptation to cortical bone loss. As bone is gradually lost from within the shafts of long bones, a smaller amount is added externally. This successful strategy uses sound engineering principles to maintain bone strength and thus, together with the low rate of loss from cortical bone, minimizes the fracture risk

tion, ceases in a young woman, there should be plenty of viable follicles left in each ovary (unless she has undergone a true premature menopause). Premenopausally, ovulation

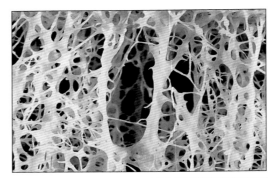

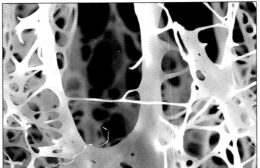

Figure 9
Adaptation to loss of trabecular bone: arcade formation in an osteoporotic vertebral body. As the transverse trabeculae become progressively thinned and disrupted, thickening of some vertical trabeculae helps to compensate for loss of their buttressing effect, but can only hold fractures at bay for a limited period if bone loss continues

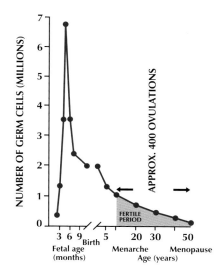

Figure 10
Profligacy in the human ovary. The numbers of germ cells peak several months before a baby girl is born. About two-thirds cease to be viable by birth, and about half of the remainder before puberty. Of the million or so germ cells that then remain, only about 400 are ever ovulated. Although 100–1000 are still present at the menopause, they no longer respond to pituitary stimulation (see *Figure 11*)

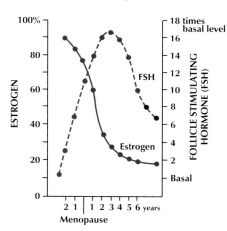

Figure 11
Hormonal changes at the menopause. Estradiol withdrawal stimulates the pituitary to produce extra FSH – up to 17 times the normal level. This attempt to restart ovulation and estradiol production provides a test for distinguishing reversible amenorrhea from the true menopause, which is invaluable in young women with a suspected premature menopause

fails because the pituitary gland is not producing sufficient follicle stimulating hormone (FSH) to bring an ovarian follicle to fruition at the mid-point of each monthly cycle.

At the menopause, whatever its timing, there will be no more than 1000 viable follicles left in either ovary, following the life-long decline in their numbers (*Figure 10*). No matter how much FSH the pituitary then produces in a vain attempt to stimulate ovulation again, the ovaries cannot respond. Far from 'pausing', natural (as opposed to HRT-induced) menstruation then comes to a final halt, more aptly described by science writer Caroline Richmond as the meno*stop*. But the pituitary tries to restart the cycle. Postmenopausally, it secretes ultra-high levels of both FSH and the luteinizing hormone (LH), which normally stimulates progesterone secretion during the second half of each cycle, in preparation for possible pregnancy. In a truly menopausal woman, the attempt is of course in vain. The demonstration of abnormally high levels of both FSH and LH, with low estradiol concentrations, does, however, provide a useful clinical test, confirming that a woman with amenorrhea is recently

postmenopausal, whatever her age (*Figure 11*). The only exceptions are postmenopausal women taking HRT – in whom FSH and LH levels decline to normal. It is not clear whether abnormally high levels of these pituitary hormones play any part in the high rates of post-menopausal bone loss.

The pattern of bone loss in Type I osteoporosis, characteristic of estradiol deficiency in postmenopausal or younger amenorrheic women, is predominantly trabecular. Only about one-third of the women with true postmenopausal osteoporosis have appreciably low cortical bone density, and this finding may be incidental, quite possibly dating (in part or whole) from a low peak bone mass 25 years or so earlier. Clinically, postmenopausal osteoporosis often presents with a wrist or other limb fracture, or with back pain, sometimes of sudden onset, caused by fractures in the trabecular bodies of one or more vertebrae. But the underlying cause often goes unrecognized at the time. Many limb fractures are initially misdiagnosed as purely accidental injuries, and the pain of vertebral fractures may be attributed to lumbago (which means little more than pain in the lower back), sciatica or a lumbar disc lesion. Two or more limb or vertebral fractures may have to occur, perhaps accompanied by thoracic kyphosis, back pain and/or loss of stature, before the true diagnosis is suspected – and even more time may elapse before it is confirmed by special investigations and treated.

Although mainly postmeno-pausal, Type I bone loss is not confined to women. A small number of men of similar age, thought to represent about 5% of cases, also suffer from osteoporosis with similar features, which may or may not be associated with testosterone deficiency.

TRANSITIONAL CHANGES

The rapid loss of trabecular bone in the early postmenopausal years is associated with high rates of bone turnover. Like the advent of estradiol at puberty, its withdrawal at the menopause precipitates a period of active remodelling at numerous sites, particularly in trabecular bone. But the bone which waxed in adolescence is now on the wane, actively acclimatizing itself to a diminished role, perhaps in prepara-tion for a quieter life. This continues for a few years after the menopause before the turnover rate falls back towards normal premenopausal levels and the rate of loss stabilizes – though with wide individual varia-tion, and at best for only 10 years' respite before the onset of the age-related changes that herald senile osteoporosis. Some women contin-ue to lose trabecular bone at an enhanced rate for a decade or more after the menopause, often with nothing more than a slight physique and an increasingly bent figure to suggest that they may be at high risk. Others may be partially protected from excessive bone loss by what is normally regarded as an adverse factor: their own obesity.

PROTECTIVE OBESITY

Osteoporosis flies in the face of contemporary wisdom about the health virtues of keeping slim. Obese women generally run a lower risk of becoming osteoporotic than their slim sisters. Their bones benefit in several distinct ways. The estro-gen, estrone, is synthesized naturally in the body fat, in proportion to its quantity: the fatter the person, the greater the amount of hormone produced. Though not as efficient as estradiol in promoting strong bones, estrone is partly converted into estradiol and does have the effect of stimulating collagen synthesis, thus contributing to the full faces and blooming complexions of many women who are overweight and helping to curb their bone loss. Carrying excess weight also helps to strengthen the bones of obese people of either sex who are physi-cally active, and their diet is of course unlikely to be deficient in vitamin D or protein, though they may lack calcium. None of this makes obesity incompatible with postmenopausal or senile osteo-porosis; it just reduces the risk. As at other ages, there are also wide, and still inexplicable, individual varia-tions in susceptibility to osteoporo-sis and in its severity, though women who have already suffered post-menopausal bone loss are inevitably at greater risk than men of the same age.

This sex difference may have been aggravated in recent years, to the further disadvantage of middle-aged women, by their husbands being advised to go on low-fat diets to lower the risk of coronary heart disease. Many wives then adopt the same diet, rather than prepare separate food. Their calcium and vitamin D intake from milk, cream, cheese and other dairy products is thus reduced, aggravating the negative calcium balance that normally follows the menopause. Fat restriction, supposed to reduce the risk of cardiovascular disease in men, may well be increasing the risk of osteoporosis in women as old age approaches.

SENILE (TYPE II) OSTEOPOROSIS

The age-related bone loss which causes senile osteoporosis is distinctive in several ways, which distinguish it from the postmenopausal type (*Table 2*). It affects both sexes, starting insidiously in the late sixties or early seventies, and appears to have multiple causes which produce characteristic changes in cortical as well as trabecular bone. About one-third of cases are male, the fact that there is a sex difference at all probably reflecting earlier events in women (chiefly lower peak bone mass, followed by postmenopausal

Table 2 Postmenopausal and senile (age-related) osteoporosis compared

	Postmenopausal (Type I)	Age-related (Type II)
Epidemiological factors		
Age (years)	55–75	> 70 (F); > 80 (M)
Sex ratio (F/M)	6 : 1	2 : 1
Bone physiology or metabolism		
Pathogenesis	Increased osteoclast activity; ↑ resorption	Decreased osteoblast activity; ↓ formation
Net bone loss	Mainly trabecular	Cortical and trabecular
Rate of bone loss	Rapid/short duration	Slow/long duration
Bone density	> 2 standard deviations below normal	Low normal (adjusted for age and sex)
Clinical signs		
Fracture sites	Vertebrae (crush), distal forearm, hip (intracapsular)	Vertebrae (multiple wedge), proximal humerus and tibia, hip (extracapsular)
Other signs	Tooth loss	Dorsal kyphosis
Laboratory values		
Serum calcium	Normal	Normal
Serum progesterone	Normal	Normal
Alkaline phosphatase	Normal (↑ with fracture)	Normal (↑ with fracture)
Urinary calcium	Increased	Normal
PTH function	Decreased	Increased
Renal conversion of 25 (OH)D to 1,25 (OH)$_2$D	Secondary decrease due to ↓ PTH	Primary decrease due to decreased responsiveness of 1-α-OH$_{ase}$
Gastrointestinal calcium absorption	Decreased	Decreased
Prevention		
High-risk patients	Estrogen or calcitonin supplementation; calcium supplementation; adequate vitamin D; adequate weight-bearing activity; minimization of associated risk factors	Calcium supplementation; adequate vitamin D; adequate weight-bearing activity; minimization of associated risk factors Bisphosphonates

loss) and their continuing estrogen lack, rather than greater female susceptibility to senile osteoporosis as such. The established condition typically presents as a hip fracture in the late seventies or eighties, involving the neck or adjacent parts of the

include dietary or metabolic deficiencies (affecting calcium, vitamin D and possibly protein), hormone (testosterone or estradiol) deficiency, lack of weight-bearing exertion to strengthen the bones, and age-related declines in calcium absorption and renal control of calcium excretion. The blood calcium is consequently low in senile (though high in

Fracture of right femoral neck. Characteristic external rotation and shortening of limb

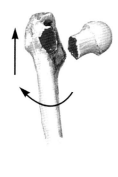

upper femur (*Figure 12*), in contrast to the vertebral and wrist fractures more characteristic of postmenopausal osteoporosis. The distinction is not complete, however. Other limb fractures are common in old age, and about 30% of patients with senile osteoporosis also have vertebral fractures, some of long-standing. But then Type II osteoporosis in the elderly of either sex is always superimposed on the sum total of all previous bone losses, cortical as well as trabecular, and can only draw on the same diminishing reserve – the peak bone mass established 40 or 50 years earlier.

postmenopausal) osteoporosis. This may then cause further bone loss, since resorption is stimulated, releasing more calcium from bone, apparently in an attempt to raise the blood level. Enhanced resorption is typically combined with low rates of bone formation, leading to incomplete infilling of resorption cavities, as in other forms of osteoporosis. The senile type is distinguished by more balanced loss of cortical as well as trabecular bone, in men as well as women.

Figure 12
Fracture of the femoral neck in old age, showing the characteristic shortening and external rotation of the affected leg – often the first signs of osteoporosis that has been silently developing for many years. It is not yet clear how much HRT or other forms of preventive therapy can reduce the risk of this common fracture, which continues to be life-threatening and potentially disabling despite major advances in its surgical repair

MULTIPLE CAUSES

The severity of senile osteoporosis depends upon the cumulative effect of all such earlier factors as well as the rate of bone loss in old age. Its multiple causes are thought to

Whether senile osteoporosis further weakens the femoral neck, sufficiently to increase the risk of fracture, is disputed. Bone density measurements reveal only small average differences (and some overlapping) between patients with femoral fractures and age-matched controls. This makes it impossible to forecast individual fracture risk at all accurately in the elderly by taking densitometry readings in the neck of the femur. By contrast, low densitometry values in the vertebral bodies are highly predictive of vertebral fractures in postmenopausal osteoporosis, enabling those at high risk to be identified in advance. Other factors may, therefore, be at least as important as bone loss in predisposing to hip fractures in senile osteoporosis. The infirmities of age are obvious candidates: failing eyesight, doddery, unstable gait (associated with arthritis, muscle weakness and/or loss of position sense), confusion, parkinsonism, slowed reactions and so forth – any or all of which may greatly increase the risks both of falling and of sustaining injuries through failure to take effective avoiding action quickly enough. But these may not be the only infirmities that threaten old bones.

LOSS OF BONE QUALITY?

The quality of bone itself appears to decline in old age. This quite probably means that the physical strength of aging bone is no longer commensurate with its mineral density. The angular, shearing forces to which the shape of the femoral neck exposes it more than any other weight-bearing bone may make it particularly prone to fracture when weakened in this way. That, together with the greater risk of old people falling heavily, could help to explain why the substantial earlier loss of bone mineral from the femoral neck in middle-aged women is not followed by a material increase in fractures, whereas much smaller additional losses in old age so often are. The degree of bone loss is not closely correlated with the fracture risk in either case. Since the weakened femoral neck rarely fractures in the fifties or sixties, the earlier bone loss may be regarded as appropriate adaptation, reducing its strength, within safe limits, to match the reduced stresses likely to be encountered. In old age, the everyday stresses on the femoral neck do not increase to strengthen it in preparation for the growing risk of falling. Quite the opposite. Activity declines, bone loss tends to accelerate, and bone quality may deteriorate.

OSTEOCYTE CHANGES

The age-related deterioration in the condition of the osteocytes and the decline in their numbers, as demonstrated by Ralis and colleagues in Cardiff over many years, seem most unlikely to be incidental findings of no pathological importance. In its simplest terms, the crucial question is whether these changes actually cause loss of bone quality or are just a feature of it. Since their severity is related to bone loss as well as age, it is tempting to assume that a complete network of osteocytes and lining cells is required for maintenance of strong bones. Any disruption of the network by cells dying or deteriorating would then impair control of bone turnover, leading to loss of bone and ultimately to a decline in the quality of what remains. There is no proof of this at present. But some such failure in senile osteoporosis seems likely to predispose to fractures in old age – and may possibly account for the rapid deterioration of osteoporosis in some younger patients, not all of them women, which cannot be explained in the present state of knowledge. It would hardly be surprising if aging bone eventually gave up the unequal struggle to control and adapt to loss of its substance, and the degenerative changes observed in the osteocytes make them the most likely candidates. Time, and further research, will show. Meanwhile, there is steadily increasing scope not only for building up the bone mass to an optimal peak, and for limiting subsequent bone loss, but also for screening programs to identify those at risk of osteoporosis, with a view to early prevention.

Bibliographical notes

Several reviews of the etiology and pathogenesis of osteoporosis have appeared recently [Raisz L.G. (1993), Local and systemic factors in the pathogenesis of osteoporosis, *World Rev. Nutr. Diet*, **72**, 92–101; Wark J.D. (1993), Osteoporosis: pathogenesis, diagnosis, prevention and management, *Baillieres Clin. Endocrinol. Metab.*, **7**, 151–81; Heaney R.P. (1993), Bone mass, nutrition, and other lifestyle factors, *Am. J. Med.*, **95 suppl. 5A**, 29S–33S; Simon L. (1993), Pathogenesis of osteoporosis, *Bull. Rheum. Dis.*, **42**, 1–3]. The distinction between postmenopausal and senile types of osteoporosis made 12 years ago [Riggs B.L. and Melton L.J. (1983), Evidence for two distinct syndromes of involutional osteoporosis, *Am. J. Med.*, **75**, 899–901] has been followed by many studies of bone loss at different stages of life [e.g. Sowers M.R. *et al.* (1993), Epidemiology of bone mass in premenopausal women, *Epidemiol. Rev.*, **15**, 374–98; Lindsay R. (1993), Pathogenesis of postmenopausal osteoporosis, *Baillieres Clin. Rheumatol.*, **7**, 499–513; Martin B. (1993), Aging and strength of bone as a structural material, *Calcif. Tissue Int.*, **53 suppl. 1**, S34–40].

Interest has recently shifted to predisposing lifestyle factors, such as dietary deficiencies [Heaney R.P. (1993), Nutritional factors in osteoporosis, *Annu. Rev. Nutr.*, **13**, 287–316; Bullamore J.R. *et al.* (1970), Effect of age on calcium absorption, *Lancet*, **2**, 535–7; Nilas, L. Calcium intake and osteoporosis, *World Rev. Nutr. Diet*, **73**, 1–26], lack of calcium and/or vitamin D [Sowers M. (1993), Epidemiology of calcium and vitamin D in bone loss, *J. Nutr.*, **123 suppl. 2**, 413–7], inadequate physical activity [Pocock N.A. *et al.* (1986), Physical fitness is a major determinant of femoral neck and lumbar spine bone mineral density, J. Clin. Invest., **78**, 618-21; Oxnard C.E. (1993), Bone and bones, architecture and stress, fossils and osteoporosis,

J. Biomech., **26 suppl. 1**, 63–79; Chesnut C.H. (1993), Bone mass and exercise, *Am. J. Med.*, **95 suppl. 5A**, 34S–36S; Snow-Harter C.M. (1994), Bone health and prevention of osteoporosis in active and athletic women, *Clin. Sports Med.*, **13**, 389–404]. Recognition of such factors can be harnessed to prevention [Anderson J.J. *et al.* (1993), Contributions of dietary calcium and physical activity to primary prevention of osteoporosis in females, *J. Am. Coll. Nutr.*, **12**, 378–83].

Increasing attention is being paid to the more profound effect of lifestyle factors that induce amenorrhea in girls [Putukian M. (1994), The female triad: Eating disorders, amenorrhea, and osteoporosis, *Med. Clin. North Am.*, **78**, 345–56; Nativ A. *et al.* (1994), The female athlete triad. The inter-relatedness of disordered eating, amenorrhea, and osteoporosis, *Clin. Sports Med.*, **13**, 405–18; Welti H. *et al.* (1992), Amenorrhoea and risk of osteoporosis in the adolescent (French), *Arch. Gynecol. Obstet.*, **252 suppl.**, S9–13; Drinkwater B.L. *et al.* (1984), Bone mineral content of amenorrhoeic and eumenorrhoeic athletes, *N. Engl. J. Med.*, **311**, 277–81]. The effects of contraception and lactation on bone density have also received attention [e.g. Mehta S. (1993), Bone loss, contraception and lactation, *Acta Obstet. Gynecol. Scand.*, **72**, 148–56], as have the normally protective effect of pregnancy and the relatively rare form of acute bone loss that it can precipitate [Reid I.R. *et al.* (1992), Pregnancy osteoporosis, *Clin. Endocrinol. (Oxf.)*, **3**, 298–303].

The adverse effect of corticosteroid therapy on bone growth and density is increasingly recognized [e.g. Olbricht T. *et al.* (1993), Corticosteroid-induced osteoporosis, *J. Intern. Med.*, **34**, 237–44; Reid I.R. (1993), Steroid osteoporosis, *Osteoporos. Int.*, **suppl. 3**, 1–6; Hosking D.J. (1993), Effects of corticosteroids on bone turnover, *Respir. Med.*, **87 suppl. A**, 15–21; Adachi J.D. *et al.* (1993), Corticosteroid-induced osteoporosis, *Semin. Arthrit, Rheum.*, **22**, 675–84; Reid I.R. *et al.* (1994), Glucocorticoid osteoporosis, *J. Asthma*, **31**, 7–18; Jenkinson T. *et al.* (1993), A reappraisal of steroid-induced osteoporosis, *Br. J. Hosp. Med.*, **50**, 472–6]. There is growing evidence that inhaled corticosteroids also affect the bones, though less severely [Jones K.S. *et al.* (1993), Osteoporosis as a result of inhaled steroids, *Ann. Pharmacother.*, **27**, 1470–2; Reid, D.M. (1993), Measurement of bone turnover and clinical investigation of osteoporosis; relevance to asthma and corticosteroid therapy, *Respir. Med.*, **87 suppl. A**, 9–14]. A good general review of the mechanisms of steroid-induced osteoporosis that appeared 5 years ago remains hard to beat, if no longer fully up to date [Lukert B.P. and Raisz L.G. (1990), Glucocorticoid-induced osteoporosis: pathogenesis and management, *Ann. Intern. Med.*, **112**, 352–64]. The many causes of 'Secondary osteoporosis' have been reviewed by I.T. Boyle 1993) [*Baillieres Clin. Rheumatol.*, **7**, 515–34].

Osteoporosis in men has been attracting greater attention [Scane A.C. *et al.* (1993), Osteoporosis in men, *Baillieres Clin. Rheumatol.*, **7**, 589–601], as have its local causes in either sex [e.g. Jones S.M. *et al.* (1993), Osteoporosis in rheumatoid arthritis, *Clin. Exp. Rheumatol.*, **11**, 557–62].

Though not wholly up-to-date, two reviews clarify the various factors (including smoking) known to influence the age at menopause [Stanford J.L. *et al.* (1987), Factors influencing the age at natural menopause, *J. Chron Dis.*, **40**, 995–1002; Ginsburg J. (1991), What determines the age at menopause? (editorial), *Br. Med. J.*, **302**, 1288–9]. Their combined effect is far too small, however, to account for a premature menopause in the teens or twenties.

Chapter 4:
Susceptibility to osteoporosis

THE KEY TO PREVENTION

Osteoporosis typically affects otherwise healthy people – just as it develops in normal bone. Many of these people could now be identified and given preventive treatment before their bones become dangerously weakened, but very few receive it. The absence of any clear-cut symptoms or clinical signs that might draw attention to their insidious bone loss not only hinders diagnosis; it means that the need for preventive measures goes unrecognized. Most postmenopausal women and members of other high-risk groups known to be susceptible to osteoporosis still have to sustain two or more fractures, typically at the wrist, spine or hip, before the diagnosis is suspected. Even then, they may not be investigated fully or given effective therapy. Yet it is never too late to prevent further bone loss and thus reduce the fracture risk – which will always continue to rise if nothing is done.

UNRECOGNIZED NEEDS

Sadly, 'nothing' still comes perilously close to the prophylactic norm, even among high-risk groups. Their needs are simply neglected. In western countries, where the risk of postmenopausal women becoming osteoporotic has received most publicity – and preventive measures could be most readily afforded – only a minority has ever taken any HRT or other drugs capable of controlling bone loss. Most of that minority will not have done so for long enough to obtain sustained protection. The 1990 prescribing figures quoted earlier suggest that little more than 1% of an estimated 7 million postmenopausal and elderly women in the United Kingdom were receiving any form of long-term preventive treatment for osteoporosis. The percentage may well be still lower among members of other high-risk groups whose proneness to osteoporosis is less well recognized – amenorrheic younger women, elderly men, alcoholics, and patients of either sex taking long-term corticosteroid therapy.

The corollary is inescapable. The vast majority, perhaps 99% or more, of those identifiable as being at risk from osteoporosis are not receiving preventive therapy at present. Among the few postmenopausal women who are taking long-term HRT for the sake of their bones, some are being treated 'blind', without assessment either of their individual need for it or of their response. With some justification, but no proof, the therapy is just assumed to be preventing bone loss. It is questionable how many of these women will continue to take HRT regularly for 10 years or more – in doses that are high enough, or with sufficiently frequent monitoring, to be sure that their bone density is being, at least, maintained.

None of the methods currently available can restore more than a small proportion of the bone already lost. Hence, the need to start preventive treatment as early as possible in those already losing bone at an accelerated rate. The 5 – 10 years' treatment often recommended for postmenopausal women represents an arbitrary minimum for worthwhile deferral of bone loss and its consequences, in relation to their average age and life expectancy. Many of them need to continue for longer, if their bones were seriously weakened before starting preventive treatment or if bone loss silently resumed, at an unacceptably high rate, after its withdrawal. Younger people with amenorrhea or taking corticosteroids often need to do so. Prone to much more protracted bone loss by virtue of their youth, they should take preventive measures, and have their efficacy monitored, for at least as long as the cause of their osteoporosis continues. This rarely happens in practice, however, any more than most elderly patients with senile osteoporosis – and therefore at remorselessly rising risk of hip fracture – receive preventive therapy for the rest of their days.

MISSED DIAGNOSES

At present, the chances of being investigated for osteoporosis and given properly monitored, sufficiently long-term preventive therapy are not much improved when a member of any of these high-risk groups sustains a fracture. The underlying diagnosis will often be missed. Even among the post-menopausal and elderly women most at risk, broken bones are usually attributed to their immediate cause, a fall or other accident, and treated accordingly – not interpreted as possible evidence of osteoporosis. Priority is understandably given to repair of the fracture. There may have been nothing beyond the age and sex of the patient and the occurrence of the fracture itself to suggest any underlying weakness of the bone. Indeed, much of the information available at the time may have been falsely reassuring.

The plain X-rays required to reveal a fracture often give a misleadingly normal picture of

Figure 1
Fractures in osteoporotic bone usually heal well, distracting attention from the weakness that contributed to them. The resorption of damaged bone is soon outpaced by the disproportionately large quantities of callus formed to repair and reinforce the whole area. The mineral content of a healing fracture therefore rises while bone loss continues elsewhere – even from the rest of the fractured bones

STAGES IN FRACTURE REPAIR

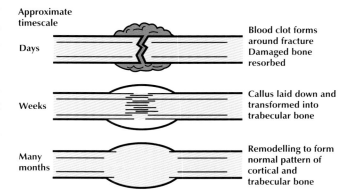

Approximate timescale

Days — Blood clot forms around fracture / Damaged bone resorbed

Weeks — Callus laid down and transformed into trabecular bone

Many months — Remodelling to form normal pattern of cortical and trabecular bone

moderately osteoporotic bone, unchanged in outline and not visibly rarefied. Nor will the course of recovery be likely to suggest anything amiss. All but the most severely osteoporotic bone usually heals quite soundly, with or without pinning or other forms of surgical fixation, and at much the same rate as normal bone. But the fact that a bone may repair itself satisfactorily, thanks to normal callus formation and subsequent remodelling, does not mean that the routine remodelling processes of resorption and formation of new bone are in balance. This may seem puzzling, since similar workforces of osteoclasts and osteoblasts are employed on both tasks. Why should they perform one so much more satisfactorily than the other?

The explanation is that osteoporotic bone retains much of its capacity for self-repair because there is a strongly *positive* imbalance between the osteoclasts which clear the site and the large quantities of callus formed (*Figure 1*). Subsequent remodelling of the callus may then run at a deficit – like the rest of an osteoporotic skeleton. In much the same way, a marginally unprofitable garage would be able to maintain the standard of its emergency repairs so long as it could call on reliable mechanics and spare parts. In neither case should small annual losses – of bone or money – affect the quality of the repair work. To find out that a garage was unprofitable, and why, one would need to inspect its books for losses in the light of the prevailing business climate. To discover whether osteoporosis has been sapping the skeleton, and understand why, it is necessary to investigate the bones for evidence of losses – in the light of the patient's age, diet, hormonal climate and so forth. Otherwise, the underlying diagnosis will be missed.

It has not proved possible to establish exactly what proportion of postmenopausal women or the elderly undergo densitometry to assess the strength of their bones after sustaining a fracture. As a rough average, no more than 5% appear to be adequately investigated within 6–12 months, and the proportion may be close to zero in some areas. Densitometry is not necessarily performed even if the bones are found to be severely weakened during operative repair of a fracture, or if its subsequent healing is impaired. These tend to be regarded as local problems, only calling for short-term solutions to heal a particular fracture, not as indications for further investigation or long-term preventive therapy. Non-surgical signs suggestive of osteoporosis also tend to be overlooked or misread in patients at risk. Backache and nerve root pain in a postmenopausal woman may be falsely attributed to a slipped disc or 'lumbago', stooping and loss of height in the elderly to becoming bent with age. Missing or misreading these warning signs leaves the high rate of bone loss that caused them to continue unchecked (*Figure 2*).

LOST OPPORTUNITIES FOR PREVENTION

If the necessary investigations belatedly reveal osteoporotic changes, much bone will already have been lost, most of it irretrievably. Yet that loss could have been curtailed, by identifying susceptible individuals in advance, and by paying more attention to early and not-so-early signs suggestive of osteoporosis, including all fractures in postmenopausal women and others recognizably at risk. Such cases should all be screened for evidence of bone loss and, if necessary, more fully investigated. Preventive therapy could then be offered to those found to have incipient or established osteoporosis, and borderline cases could be followed up to detect any future deterioration in good time. These are strictly practicable aims, for which the need is clear and the necessary technical advances have been made in recent years. They should now be universally, not haphazardly, implemented.

The effectiveness of the various diagnostic and therapeutic means required to combat osteoporosis has been amply demonstrated in clinical trials. They have yet to be brought together in a comprehensive scheme for large-scale prevention among the population as a whole. This chapter argues that they should be – and puts forward a tentative plan. The following two chapters take up the theme, with details of the diagnostic techniques and drug treatments now available for the purpose. With no prospect of

anything like a vaccine capable of giving lifelong protection, the prevention of excessive bone loss in adult life demands a long-term strategy. It should start, not belatedly at the menopause, but in earliest childhood, if not before birth. Comprehensive prevention of this kind would necessarily fall into two distinct phases, reflecting the natural history of bone's development and subsequent decline:

General prophylactic measures in babies, children, adolescents and young adults, concentrating on teenage girls, with the aim of building up the peak bone mass to its full potential by the late twenties, and

Screening of postmenopausal women and other adults at risk, to identify those who have a low bone density and/or high rates of bone loss, so that they can be fully investigated and, if necessary, given long-term preventive therapy.

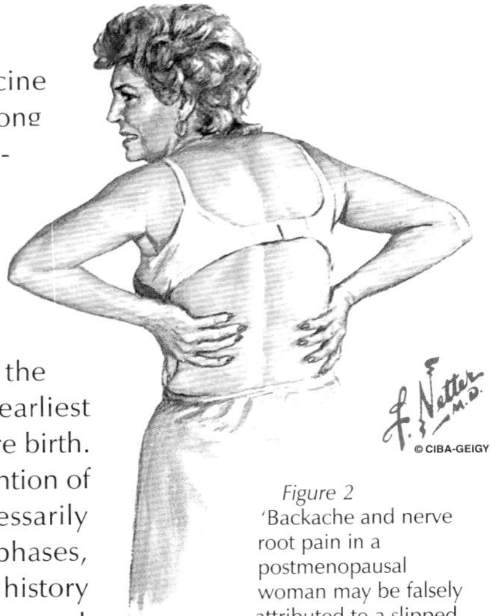

Figure 2
'Backache and nerve root pain in a postmenopausal woman may be falsely attributed to a slipped disc or lumbago...' Such warning signs of vertebral fracture are often preceded by characteristic postural changes, as shown here. Misreading them leaves bone loss to continue unchecked – or even exacerbated by the bed rest commonly recommended for acute back pain

Table 1 Building strong bones – the first stage in preventing osteoporosis

What young bones need to attain their full potential

- Well-balanced diet, containing adequate calcium, vitamin D, and protein
- Regular physical exertion to stress the bones throughout childhood and adolescence
- Puberty at normal age, followed by regular menstruation and estradiol secretion in girls, and normal testosterone levels in boys
- Absence of adverse influences, including
  - Amenorrhea, only in girls
  - Calcium deficiency, especially in adolescent girls
  - Cigarette smoking, only in girls
  - Corticosteroid therapy
  - Genetic defects (e.g. osteogenesis imperfecta)

All such factors are cumulative – for better or worse – in determining the peak bone mass achieved in early adult life

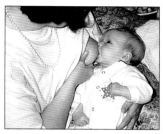

Figure 3
For optimal development, a baby's bones need adequate quantities of calcium, vitamin D and protein – normally supplied by breast milk or recognized substitutes. A milk-based diet that satisfies a baby's appetite and produces normal weight gain should not require supplements (except possibly of vitamins C and D), but breast-feeding mothers may need extra calcium and vitamin D to prevent depletion of their own bones

Figure 4
The popularity of baby foods containing cereals, vegetable purees and fruit juices – all relatively low in calcium – may mean that some babies now receive too little milk after weaning from breast or bottle. If this results in deficiency of calcium, and quite probably of vitamin D and protein, bone development could be restricted at this early age, perhaps diminishing the peak bone mass and thus predisposing to osteoporosis later in life

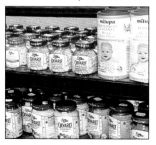

PROPHYLAXIS IN CHILDHOOD

The general measures required to build strong bones are simple in themselves and readily summarized (*Table 1*). Those appropriate to all mothers and children – adequate calcium and vitamin D, plus regular exercise to stress the skeleton – could be publicized in the mass media as general health advice, as well as being recommended in antenatal and children's clinics, by school medical services, and in general practitioners' surgeries. They are plainly of special importance in girls and in any children of either sex who are recognizably predisposed to osteoporosis later in life. Evidence of some predisposing factors may already be identifiable at birth. There would be four, for example, in a baby *girl*, born to *white or oriental parents*, of *slight physique*, who has a *family history of osteoporosis*.

How such traits predispose to osteoporosis, whether they are genetically or environmentally determined, and whether they operate by lowering the peak bone mass or by raising the rates of bone loss later in adult life, makes little difference to the preventive measures required. In either case, their aim during childhood and adolescence is to achieve the highest possible bone mass, both by creating optimal conditions for development and by minimizing any adverse influences, such as calcium deficiency or corticosteroid therapy.

Maintaining milk consumption

In infancy, when it is not desirable (or necessary) to stress the skeleton beyond a baby's normal attempts to sit up, crawl, and start to walk, breast milk (*Figure 3*) or substitutes will normally provide sufficient supplies of protein, calcium and vitamin D. A greater risk of deficiency arises after weaning, from breast or bottle. The popularity of baby foods containing cereals, vegetable purees and fruit juices (*Figure 4*) may mean that some babies now receive little milk – too little to satisfy the high demands for calcium and vitamin D created by rapid growth during the first year or more of life. Milk consumption should, therefore, be maintained when other foods are introduced. Intolerance is fortunately rare at this age, but should always be taken seriously, especially in baby girls. Cow's milk may only need to be adequately watered down and sugared to become acceptable. Alternatively, other types (e.g. goat's), milk products (such as dried milk or yoghurt), soya 'milk', or even calcium preparations as such may be better tolerated. Green vegetables are poor substitutes, most unlikely to be digestible in the quantities required for a baby (or older child) to absorb enough calcium for optimal bone development.

During early childhood, when calcium demand levels off, milk intolerance becomes a little more frequent, largely due to the development of lactase deficiency in a few children of European (and most of oriental) origin. The digestive disturbance caused by the unchanged milk sugar, lactose, may then be misdiagnosed as a food allergy, with the implication that all milk and related products must be totally avoided. In reality, lactase-deficient children and adults can safely be given as much milk as they will tolerate (often a cupful, spread over the day), supplemented by cheese or yoghurt (in which the lactose has been predigested by bacteria) and other calcium-rich foods to make up the deficit.

Corticosteroids in childhood and adolescence

The bones of children with disabling complaints like juvenile arthritis, which may restrain growth and severely restrict the exertion required for building strong bones, are doubly at risk if they need long-term treatment with systemic corticosteroids (*Figure 5*). Adverse effects on the growth and ultimate strength of bone can be limited, but not wholly eliminated, by the usual practice of carefully controlling the dosage. Impairment of calcium absorption may be slightly alleviated, but not wholly overcome, by giving regular supplements, though this is not always done, even for young patients on long-term corticosteroid therapy.

Calcium absorption is so easily inhibited by corticosteroids, as noted earlier, that the small amounts swallowed by asthmatic children, taking minimal doses by inhalation alone, are sufficient to impair bone

mineralization. Although the detailed management of such problems lies outside the scope of this book, the need for special precautions ought to be more generally appreciated in children receiving long-term corticosteroid therapy in any form – by mouth, inhaled, or applied to largish areas of skin. At present, the failure of children on systemic therapy to attain full stature is regarded as a regrettable but unavoidable side-effect of essential treatment, whereas their corresponding failure to attain a satisfactory peak bone mass tends to be overlooked altogether. Both questions deserve more attention from clinicians and researchers if the adverse effects of corticosteroids on bone development are to be reduced in future. The appreciable numbers of children and teenagers unfortunate enough to have chronic conditions requiring long-term corticosteroid treatment deserve to be relieved of the additional, long-term threat to their bones.

ADOLESCENCE AND AFTER

Following the steadier progress and more modest dietary demands of childhood, the acquisition of bone becomes critical again when the growth spurt of puberty pushes

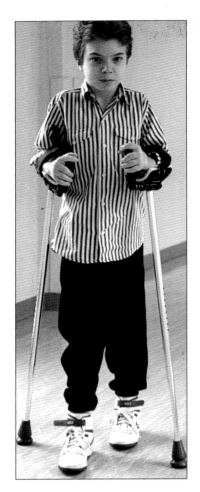
Figure 5
Growth may be doubly restricted in conditions such as juvenile polyarthritis – both by the disease itself and by the long-term corticosteroid therapy required to control it. The resulting shortness of stature is always a matter for concern, but any associated diminution of the bone mass tends to be overlooked. Long-term prevention of osteoporosis calls for close attention to such risks, particularly in girls

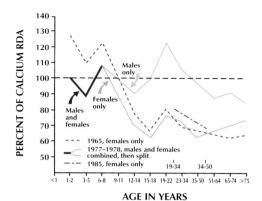

Figure 6
'To prevent osteoporosis later in life, teenagers in general, and girls in particular, need to drink more milk, eat more calcium-rich foods and undertake more physical exercise than is now customary ...' From late childhood onwards, females fall far below the recommended daily allowance (RDA) of calcium, indicated by the 100% line

calcium demand to its highest levels. Assuming that the advent of the sex hormones runs to time, it is the calcium intake during adolescence which mainly determines whether that demand is fully satisfied, enabling the bone mass to build up at an optimum rate. But most teenagers grow up without ever knowing that they had – and all-too-often missed – the last great opportunity to influence their bone mass for the better.

To prevent osteoporosis later in life, teenagers in general, and girls in particular, need to drink more milk, eat more calcium-rich foods (*Figure 6*), and undertake more physical exertion than is now customary in this age group. Adolescent girls also need to avoid smoking, and thus lowering the activity of their own estradiol, if their bones are to reach their full potential. But nobody tells them these things. That is also true of the girls at greatest risk, and therefore most in need of preventive measures: those in their teens and twenties whose puberty is delayed or who develop persistent amenorrhea after starting to menstruate normally.

Amenorrhea and estrogen deficiency

Whatever the underlying cause of amenorrhea – from endocrine and gynecological disorders, to undue slimness, excessive physical training, or heroin addiction (as discussed in Chapter 2) – it would cause most teenage girls to seek medical advice. Yet few ever learn about its ill effects on bone development. Doctors seldom warn them (if they realize themselves) that the associated estrogen deficiency will permanently reduce their bone mass. Consequently, girls with amenorrhea have no way of knowing that they may be in negative calcium balance – actually losing bone at this crucial age when they should still be building it up – and are thus deprived of the opportunity to do anything about it while there is still time. If regular menstruation cannot be established, these girls need replacement estrogens as much as any post-menopausal woman – and more than most. Their 'postmenopausal' bone loss has started 30 – 40 years prematurely . . .

Testosterone deficiency in boys

The long-term risk is also extended in teenage boys who are testosterone deficient for any reason. Delayed puberty, with growth and development of facial and pubic hair lagging behind their peers are the most frequent warning signs. Endocrine disorders apart, undescended testes are the commonest cause, because they are unable to secrete testosterone at body temperature. The sexual and physical development associated with puberty cannot take place until the testes descend into the cooler scrotum, whether naturally or by medical or surgical intervention. This will usually be all that is required for testosterone secretion to start. But long-term testosterone replacement therapy should be considered if blood levels remain low.

Without replacement therapy, the few boys who are testosterone-deficient and the much larger number of estradiol-deficient girls will not attain their potential bone mass. Achieving it must be the aim of all preventive measures, general and specific, during the first three decades of life. As matters stand at present, the whole question of identifying those who may fail to do so when they have the opportunity – and are thus predisposed to osteoporosis later in life – almost always goes by default.

GETTING THE PREVENTIVE MESSAGE ACROSS TO TEENAGERS

While it is reasonably clear what general preventive measures are advisable in childhood and adolescence, getting today's teenagers to adopt them may be quite another matter. At present, mothers and younger children would probably be the main beneficiaries of health advice on building strong bones. It may be harder to change the eating and behavioral habits of independent-minded adolescents. Dire warnings of what may happen to the bones of some of them – in the infi-

nite remoteness of middle age – would almost certainly go unheeded. Knowing about the risk of lung cancer and heart disease through smoking seems to have done less to discourage it among teenage girls than in any other sector of the population – and they are the group most in need of strong bones. More immediate, positive advice about giving their sex hormones a chance and their children a good start in life just might prove more effective.

Puppies take precedence

Sales of dog food have long been buoyed up by advertising which uses enthusiastic, cheerful slogans to convey positive messages about the value of good food and dietary additives in 'promoting health', 'building strong bones', and 'prolonging active life'. The messages would be equally appropriate for human adolescents. They may well be more acceptable than those of doleful doctors condemning junk food (whatever that is supposed to be) and crying woe over its alleged ill effects. The vets are also a step ahead in recommending routine supplements of calcium, phosphates and vitamin D to promote bone growth in puppies and kittens. Because they grow much faster than children, demand is higher, for a relatively short period. But cats and dogs live for a much shorter time than humans, experience no sudden withdrawal of hormones – unless castrated, and are much less likely to develop osteoporosis, even when they have been. If strong bones are important in young animals, they are doubly so in young men or, more specifically, women.

A bottle a day

To date, only milk has been at all widely publicized as being good for human bones, and then without any stress on the special needs of teenage girls. The total consumption of fresh milk has been falling for the past few decades in many western countries, and it would be astonishing if the young of both sexes had not shared in this widespread trend. Their reduced intake may be partly responsible for the decline in sales – and not entirely from their own choice. In the UK, for instance, milk had long been supplied free to all schoolchildren until it was withdrawn in the early 1970s, as being no longer necessary. The needs of growing bones were almost lost from sight in the political furore this provoked, and have received little public attention ever since. Perhaps these needs could best be satisfied by promoting the merits of milk for children of all ages, coupled with flashy marketing of milk shakes, yoghurts and cheeses as cheap, nutritious and, above all, trendy convenience foods for teenagers.

'Milka-Cola' – the drink of tomorrow?

The idea of something to live for here and now – to make you fitter and more attractive – may well be a better way to encourage healthier eating and more active exercise than the doom-laden warnings of much conventional health education. The teens are more a time for risk-taking than cautious precautions against future ills – even if the threat is more immediate, like that of AIDS. More distant threats are barely perceived. Soft-drinks advertising provides a striking example of what optimistic publicity can do, even for a product of no particular nutritional value. Coca-Cola, which long predates the invention of the 'teenager', has managed to build up its position as the most fashionable adolescent drink in each succeeding generation for over 100 years. It has also attracted major rivals with remarkably similar products, and spread the message around the globe. If the same could be done for a milk drink, much osteoporosis would be prevented at no cost to health services.

Towards peak bone mass

Growth ceases earlier in girls, restricting the time they have to build up the peak bone mass, compared with boys. Dietary calcium requirements then fall quite sharply in both sexes, but remodelling should continue to run at a small annual profit until the peak bone mass is reached. For that profit to be optimal, the bones need to be sustained both by normal sex hormone levels and by adequate calcium intake, so that they stay in positive balance. Building up the bone mass to its peak calls for more persistent implementation of preventive measures than either doctors or patients have been accustomed to in any existing field of preventive medicine. To retain the bone so painstakingly acquired in youth calls for a corresponding degree of sustained and close attention throughout adult life, but more selectively.

ADULTS AT RISK

By about the 30th birthday, when the peak bone mass has been passed – all unwittingly, by both men and women – the focus of prevention switches from maximizing the development of bone in all young people to minimizing its loss in older ones, with the emphasis on those at special risk. Many of the predisposing factors present in youth continue to operate. But now they accelerate loss of bone, instead of hindering its formation, and some new factors come into play, notably aging. Calcium plays a less prominent part in determining the strength of adult bones, though it is obviously necessary for the diet to contain at least the minimum required to maintain the bone mineral, which by no means all adult diets achieve. The sex hormones continue to be the dominant factor, in men as well as women, determining whether the remodelling process runs at minimal deficit – acceptable even in the long term – or accelerates, sometimes to intolerably high rates of bone loss.

All the genetic and environmental influences which predispose to osteoporosis, by impairing the development of bone, or contributing to its subsequent loss, are invariably cumulative in their adverse effects (*Table 2*). It is their sum total, set against any favorable factors, often

extending over half a century or more, which determines both the bone mass at any one time and whether bone loss will simply continue at an acceptably low rate or eventually culminate in significant osteoporosis. The causes of osteoporosis listed in Table 2 are therefore the targets for prevention.

As middle-age approaches, and estrogen levels begin to decline in normally menstruating women, the identification of high-risk individuals, who may be in need of preventive measures, becomes more pressing. Yet nothing draws direct attention to the risk. Amenorrhea in women, testosterone deficiency in men, and corticosteroid therapy in either sex – the three most common causes of accelerated bone loss in the thirties and forties – are seldom regarded as indications for densitometry or preventive therapy. The fact that any of the three enhances the risks of postmenopausal and/or senile osteoporosis is not yet generally recognized either, because there is nothing to link earlier events with bone loss that only becomes apparent 20 or 30 years later.

Table 2 Controlling bone loss – the second stage in preventing osteoporosis
Major targets for prevention, all cumulative in effect
Estrogen deficiency   • amenorrhea, polycystic ovaries, premature/surgical or natural menopause   **Testosterone deficiency**   • undescended testes, testicular fibrosis, etc.   **Calcium/vitamin D deficiency**   • dietary, malabsorption   **Corticosteroid therapy**   • long-term, especially high dosage, also inhaled, cutaneous, etc.   **Lack of weight-bearing exertion**   • inactivity, bed-rest, disability, weightlessness   **Effects of aging**   • reductions in activity, sex hormones, calcium and vitamin D absorption; changes in metabolism and bone
For correctable causes of secondary osteoporosis, see Table 1 in Chapter 3

HORMONE REPLACEMENT THERAPY FOR THE BONES

The first event in the insidious course of osteoporosis at all likely to be recognized as a causative factor – and thus trigger an appropriate preventive response – is the menopause itself. But, despite the growing public interest in HRT for the relief of menopausal symptoms, only a minority of postmenopausal women are yet aware of any risk to their bones. Only a few of those who do start taking it understand how long they need to continue, to prevent osteoporosis. And very few postmenopausal women taking HRT, or their own doctors, are aware that its withdrawal will inevitably precipitate several years of accelerated bone loss. This mimics the first 2 or 3 years of high losses, associated with high rates of bone remodelling, which follow the cessation of natural estradiol secretion at the menopause. The characteristic relapse, from breaking even or gaining bone on treatment to losing it quite rapidly after withdrawal (*Figure 7*) has been demonstrated in many of the published clinical trials, which have established HRT as the single most effective means of preventing postmenopausal bone loss. Yet the importance of maintaining preventive therapy regularly for at least 5 – 10 years after the menopause –

Figure 7
Accelerated bone loss follows estrogen withdrawal at any age – whether in young women who cease to menstruate, after the menopause, or (as here, in the radius), when HRT is discontinued. Two years' painstaking gain in bone mass while taking HRT may be lost within a year of its withdrawal. Hence the importance of maintaining regular preventive therapy for at least 5–10 years, and continuing to monitor the bone density after its withdrawal

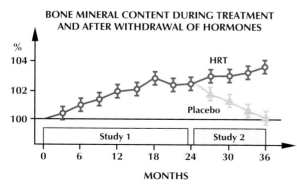

so as to protect the bones from further loss (and the arteries from atherosclerosis) – has scarcely begun to be reflected in prescribing.

A convincing decline in the total number of osteoporotic fractures in the postmenopausal population (as opposed to a study group) is not likely to become detectable until a quarter of the women whose bones are at risk take it regularly, in adequate dosage, for at least 5 years. Even if prescribing of long-term HRT were to multiply several times overnight, it might still take another decade or more before fracture rates in postmenopausal women began to decline overall. Another two decades would then have to pass before women who had taken HRT in their fifties and sixties could show any appreciable reduction in the number of fractures caused by senile osteoporosis – when they reached their seventies and eighties.

But can we afford to wait? Ought the prevention of osteoporosis not be made the subject of major public health campaigns before there is absolute proof that present methods can lower overall fracture rates in old age? Without such campaigns, prevention would be confined to limited numbers of largely self-selected postmenopausal women, not necessarily at high risk. Perhaps the key question is not whether we can afford to wait, but whether delay in getting prevention to those in greatest need is any longer tolerable – with an aging population, increasingly at risk of fractures and other complications.

WAITING FOR WHAT?

To date, the wider use of HRT or other drugs to prevent osteoporosis seems to have been hindered mainly by ignorance and caution – among doctors as well as potential patients. Despite growing interest in osteoporosis, ignorance is still widespread about its nature and long-term consequences, about who is at risk and why, about early detection of bone loss, and about the indications for, and most appropriate methods of, investigation and preventive treatment. Clarification of these practical questions may not wholly overcome other reservations. Many apparently healthy people are understandably cautious about being turned into patients, with the aim of reducing a long-term risk of little immediate concern to them or, indeed, their doctors.

The concept of giving active drugs over long periods for prevention rather than the treatment of existing disease is still unfamiliar in itself. That may contribute to an understandable fear of side-effects, especially when coupled with doubts about the need for preventive therapy or its necessarily prolonged duration. In particular, it may underlie the common but largely unjustified belief that long-term HRT increases the risk of breast cancer (an important question discussed in Chapter 6). Many postmenopausal women also have reservations about the 'unnaturalness' of taking replacement hormones, about the inconvenience of artificially induced menstruation (just

when they thought they had got rid of the 'curse' for good), and about the discomfort and niggling anxiety provoked by other side-effects such as breast tenderness.

Many general practitioners share their reservations, while experts on osteoporosis have yet to agree on the best preventive strategy. Some favor a 'population approach' to all postmenopausal women, on the questionable grounds that it would be impractical and/or too costly to identify individuals at high risk. But this is open to many objections. It would impose treatment on many women who did not really need it, while missing all the other susceptible groups, notably younger amenorrheic women, patients of both sexes receiving corticosteroid therapy, heavy drinkers and elderly men. It also raises serious doubts about compliance. Would apparently healthy women, identified only as members of a high-risk group, with no symptoms to relieve, really be willing to take supposedly preventive measures on trust for years on end, when the need had not been individually demonstrated, the treatment might have serious side-effects, and its beneficial action on bone was not being monitored?

The answer seems obvious, yet various schemes of this general type have been put forward in recent years. Some have proposed that all postmenopausal women should take calcium and/or milk supplements and regular exercise for the rest of their days, but the necessary degree of compliance sustained over several decades of declining mental and physical powers can hardly be expected. Others have suggested that estrogen replacement therapy should be given to all post-menopausal women for 5 or 10 years, or even indefinitely. While this should prove far more effective in preventing bone loss, the long-term use of HRT in unselected patients without individual monitoring is open to serious question. At worst, it might fail to control the bone loss it was supposed to be preventing, delay recognition of the fact, and cause serious side-effects. Prevention of osteoporosis calls for an altogether more rigorous approach.

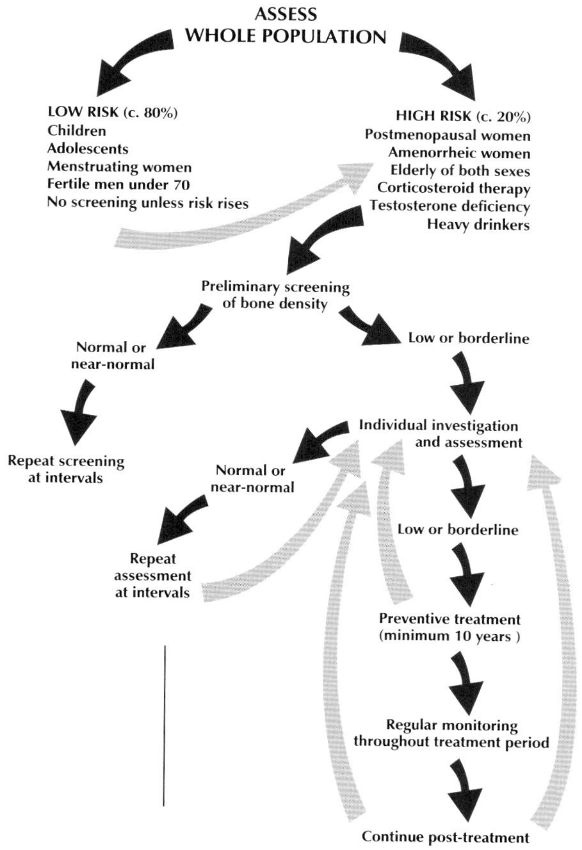

No prophylactic plan requiring long-term therapy with potent drugs could safely be based on anything but individual assessment, prescribing and follow-up throughout the treatment period, however large the numbers concerned. To handle all the people recognizably at risk from osteoporosis – approaching 20% of the population in industrialized countries – their huge numbers would need to be cut down in several stages, on something like the lines indicated in *Figure 8*. But it would not be possible simply to reassure those not found to need further investigation or treatment – and simply discharge them. Most of them would, after all, still be at increasing risk from progressive bone loss. To cope with the insidious, persistent and yet unpredictable nature of osteoporosis, with its variability both between individuals and over time, the necessary monitoring and preventive measures would have to be sustained indefinitely, not only to:

Screen the steady flow of recently postmenopausal women and others newly identified as being at risk, and to

Monitor those already taking preventive therapy, but also to

Recheck all the remainder, previously on treatment or not yet considered to need it, at appropriate intervals.

Figure 8
A possible approach to population screening and prevention of osteoporosis. The principal aim is to identify those potentially at risk – because they are postmenopausal, elderly, amenorrheic or taking corticosteroid therapy – and then screen their bones to reveal those who need preventive therapy because their bone densities are low or below the 'fracture threshold'. All would need to be re-checked at appropriate intervals – to confirm the efficacy of treatment or reassess the need for it

ASSESS WHOLE POPULATION

LOW RISK (c. 80%)
Children
Adolescents
Menstruating women
Fertile men under 70
No screening unless risk rises

HIGH RISK (c. 20%)
Postmenopausal women
Amenorrheic women
Elderly of both sexes
Corticosteroid therapy
Testosterone deficiency
Heavy drinkers

Preliminary screening of bone density

Normal or near-normal

Low or borderline

Repeat screening at intervals

Individual investigation and assessment

Normal or near-normal

Low or borderline

Repeat assessment at intervals

Preventive treatment (minimum 10 years)

Regular monitoring throughout treatment period

Continue post-treatment

Since there is no preventive therapy capable of conquering osteoporosis once and for all, either in the population as a whole or in individuals at risk, the task would be never-ending. Any such scheme would therefore have to be constantly reviewed, and modified when necessary, not only to take advantage of the diagnostic and therapeutic advances certain to continue in the field, but also to learn from its own accumulating experience. In this way, a sufficiently large-scale scheme should also be able to monitor several aspects of its own effectiveness, in reducing the numbers of fractures and other complications attributed to osteoporosis and in saving the costs of caring for them.

This need be no distant dream. The necessary technical advances have already been made in recent years, fully evaluated by research, and tried and tested in practice. The only ingredient now missing is the collective will – medical, political and financial – to set up and fund major projects for the prevention of osteoporosis. But they would obviously have to compete with other projects for priority. Here there is a danger that osteoporosis might become a perennial poor relation, never dramatic enough to bring it to the top of the list of official priorities for health budgeting. This obstacle seems likely to be overcome by popular demand.

If enough postmenopausal women and others, who can readily identify themselves as being at risk, press for screening tests, both individually and collectively, then the demand for diagnosis and preventive treatment will quickly overwhelm existing facilities and lead to their expansion. Television 'commercials' advising post-menopausal women to seek screening may be having just that effect since the National Osteoporosis Society started screening them in the UK, in 1993 (*Figure 9*).

INDIVIDUALS AT RISK

Consideration of no more than six factors – age, sex, menstrual status, corticosteroid therapy, undescended testes or other evidence of male infertility, and heavy drinking – should enable most of those at risk to distinguish themselves from the remaining 80% or so of the population. A simple questionnaire based on these major categories could easily be self-administered. Together with a check-list of other predisposing factors for osteoporosis, like those listed in Table 2, it should enable most if not all of the 20% or more of the population at risk to be identified. The second step in the proposed scheme – screening bone density – should allow the numbers to be whittled down further. Of the densitometry techniques to be described in the next chapter, simplified forms of single-photon absorptiometry (SPA), for the forearm bones, and dual X-ray absorptiometry (DXA), for the hip and/or lumbar spine, are at present most suitable for screening purposes. Either can be performed quickly without inconveniencing the patient and at reasonable cost. Until

Figure 9
The first TV 'commercial' advising postmenopausal women to have their bones screened for osteoporosis – a promising initiative by the National Osteoporosis Society in the United Kingdom, intended to identify women at high risk. Before its first screening, in north-east England in spring 1993, agreement was reached with local radiologists and health authorities, to ensure that they were prepared to cope with the anticipated demand

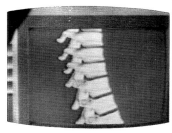

'After menopause you could lose...

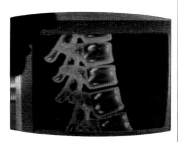

up to 30% of your bone mass to osteoporosis before you even know...

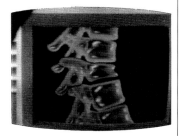

you have it'

more experience of their significance was acquired, low or borderline readings of bone density in these screening tests might need to be followed by full-scale densitometry and perhaps by other investigations to determine the severity of bone loss at other sites and to estimate its rate. In the future, with accumulating experience, it should become possible to devise screening procedures which could serve as the sole indication for preventive therapy, and for monitoring its efficacy, thus reducing the need for more detailed, time-consuming, and costly investigation.

PRESCRIBING FOR PREVENTION

A decision to start preventive therapy would rest very largely on the mineral content of bones at vulnerable sites, typically the forearm bones and lumbar spine in postmenopausal women and the hip region in the elderly. Whether caused by recent bone loss, by a low peak bone mass earlier in adult life, or by a combination of both, low bone density itself is the key factor – highly predictive of fracture risk in the forearm and lumbar spine though less so in the femoral neck (*Figure 10*).

The aim of the various types of preventive therapy now available is broadly the same: to reduce the risk of fracture by limiting further bone loss and building up the bone mass as much as may be possible. This calls for individual prescribing, to match drug and dosage to each patient's needs, including her (or his)

personal preferences. Explaining the need for long-term preventive therapy, and the pros and cons of different methods, would be vital in securing the patient's wholehearted agreement and collaboration. Without that, compliance with many years' preventive therapy could hardly be expected. Of the drugs now shown to be effective in controlling bone loss, HRT would clearly be appropriate for most amenorrheic and postmenopausal women, the others being more often required in men, in the elderly of either sex, and for some patients on corticosteroids. Details of the drugs themselves, the indications for their use, and their modes of action are outlined in Chapter 6. Between them, they should now enable osteoporosis to be controlled (whatever its cause) and often reversed to some extent in virtually every individual at risk.

PROS AND CONS OF PROPHYLAXIS

Osteoporosis now presents more favorable opportunities for large-scale prophylaxis than many other serious conditions, including heart disease and most forms of cancer. Nearly all of those at risk can be identified in advance by factors known to cause bone loss (sex hormone deficiency, aging, corticosteroid therapy, excessive drinking and so forth). These can be appropriately referred to as *predisposing* or *causative* factors, because they represent firm evidence of causation, in contrast to the *risk* factors, much in vogue for coronary heart disease and other conditions of complex and, as yet, uncertain cause. The difference has a crucial bearing on the rationale and effectiveness of preventive measures.

Strictly speaking, a risk factor is anything at all – past or present, genetic or environmental – more often present in people who develop a particular disease (or other pathological event) than in the population as a whole. It is not a known cause of the disease in question, though it might prove to be one. Identifying people with risk factors is, therefore, of limited and uncertain preventive value. Modifying risk factors whose causative role has not been proved is a lottery, which may or may not reduce the risk of developing the disease in question. Attempts to curb coronary heart disease by reducing acknowledged risk factors, like raised blood lipids or high blood pressure, seem to be foundering partly for these reasons, partly for two others. A supposedly preventive measure (such as low-fat diet) may not be strictly adhered to, or may (like lowering blood pressure as a means of preventing heart attacks) be relatively ineffective in itself. Reversing a proven causative factor like estradiol deficiency by giving HRT to a postmenopausal woman is totally different. It comes much closer to specific correction of a deficiency disease, by reversing the adverse effects of estradiol deficiency on the bones and cardiovascular system, in particular, for as long as the treatment is continued. HRT is also the most effective way to reduce the risk of coronary heart disease in postmenopausal women – probably more effective than modification of all other coronary risk factors, including smoking, combined.

Screening – a worthwhile procedure?

Screening for osteoporosis should have similar advantages over some of its more fashionable applications – in the early detection, and hoped-for prevention, of breast (*Figure 11*) and cervical cancers, for example. Screening is so obviously desirable that few question its value. Its aim is deceptively simple – to detect potentially serious conditions at a presymptomatic stage in apparently healthy people. But the benefits, or otherwise, of screening programs depend on several assumptions which may or may not be justified. The condition in question must be detectable at a stage when it is not yet causing symptoms, and no abnormal signs would betray its presence on ordinary clinical examination. The disease process must then obligingly pause (or advance in slow motion) for long enough to give routine screening tests, performed every few years at most, a fair chance of detecting its presence 'early', i.e. before it has progressed to a more severe or irreversible phase.

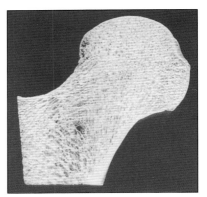

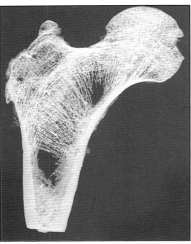

Figure 10
Osteoporosis in the head, neck and upper shaft of femur from an otherwise fit woman in her early seventies (*below*), compared with the denser trabeculation still present in a woman of 45 (*above*). The typical areas of bone loss, including Ward's triangle, clearly predispose to fracture, yet low mineral density in the femoral neck is a relatively poor predictor of fracture in the elderly – complicating the question of prevention in old age

Not all serious diseases behave in this obliging fashion. Few pause for administratively convenient 5-yearly check-ups to catch them early. Others present with presymptomatic signs suggestive of early disease, which may resolve spontaneously. And then, of course, the preventive effect of all screening depends on the existence of curative or corrective treatment, more effective in early than in established disease, and on this treatment being available promptly when required. As with risk factors, too much has been expected of screening programs in which these criteria have not been satisfied. Pre- and postmenopausal osteoporosis is unusual in being able to satisfy them all, and this may well prove to be equally true of bone loss associated with testosterone deficiency in men.

Corticosteroid-induced and senile osteoporosis

The value of screening for corticosteroid-induced and senile osteoporosis may, however, be rather more questionable for different reasons. Although screening tests should have no difficulty in detecting low bone density in patients receiving long-term corticosteroids, the efficacy of different kinds of preventive therapy has yet to be firmly established.

In senile osteoporosis, the questionable correlation between densitometry findings and fracture risk in the neck of the femur casts doubt on the feasibility of detecting elderly people at special risk of hip fracture – and, therefore, on the value of preventive therapy. While much can now be done, and should be done more widely, to combat senile osteoporosis as such, it may be better treated pre-emptively, at least in women. HRT offers the best prospect at present. By preventing earlier bone loss, it will probably prove to defer the onset of severe osteoporosis for long enough to reduce the risk of hip or other fractures in elderly women – though not eliminate it altogether. Old people will still be prone to fall and break their bones, however strong.

Figure 11
Women are being increasingly screened for breast cancer with the aim of reducing the mortality by facilitating early diagnosis and treatment, though the benefits have yet to be firmly established. A sound case can be made for the early diagnosis and preventive therapy of osteoporosis, and high-risk individuals are easier to identify, yet bone screening is much less readily available

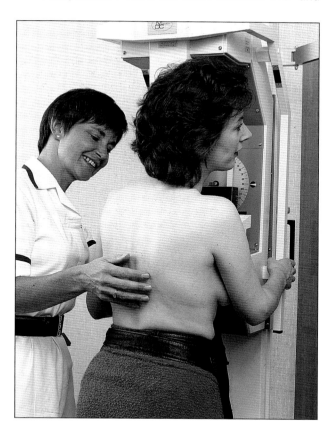

Cost effectiveness of preventive therapy

The cost of even a limited preventive program would be formidable because of the numbers at risk. Postmenopausal and elderly women now make up over 20% of the population in industrialized countries. Together with the smaller numbers of younger women at risk, they must total at least 7 million in the UK alone. At a rock bottom cost of about £25 a head for simple densitometry screening on a large scale, the initial expense of a comprehensive preventive program could hardly be less than £250 million, without allowing for its administration or for further investigation, treatment costs or follow-up. The expense would not be incurred all at once, however. Initial screening would have to be spread over at least a decade, to cover the entire population at risk, before it could settle down to routine screening of newly menopausal women and others freshly at risk, plus follow-up of those screened previously, whether receiving preventive therapy or not.

The running costs of a monitored program on these lines need not be unreasonable in relation to those of treatment and after-care of osteoporotic fractures and their sequelae. The least expensive forms of HRT cost only £15–20 a year for each patient; although the most expensive types of preventive therapy run to several times as much, lower prices could no doubt be negotiated for a large-scale national scheme.

Suppose that only 20–25% of those identified as being at risk, i.e. a total of about 2 million in the UK, were found to have a low bone density needing HRT or other drugs, their basic cost could be as little as £40 million per annum. Allowing for some more expensive preparations, together with administrative expenses and the cost of rechecking the bone density – initially, after 1 year, say, and then every 5 years on average – the total running costs might be kept below £150 million per annum. When set against the 1992 estimate of over £600 million for annual hospital costs of hip fracture alone, this suggests that preventive therapy should prove cost-effective in the long run, even if hip fractures were cut by less than half – as well as relieving much suffering and reducing the many deaths and disabilities that follow fractures in the elderly.

FUTURE EXPECTATIONS

There are, of course, a few catches in this persuasive argument. While preventive therapy for osteoporosis should save money in the long run, assuming it fulfils its high promise by reducing the number of hip fractures, substantial savings in treatment costs could hardly be expected until a large-scale scheme had been under way for 20 years or more. Any unexpected difficulties might defer the anticipated savings even longer. There is no precedent for a scheme involving such huge numbers, or for such a protracted period, in any other field of preventive medicine. It is impossible to foresee what organizational and personal problems might arise from the need to sustain the preventive impetus, year in, year out, throughout the at-risk population, for at least a decade and often for the rest of their lives. If administrative difficulties can be overcome, and individual motivation maintained, the overall balance of benefits over side-effects and costs should eventually be favorable – perhaps even releasing substantial medical resources and funding for other purposes.

There is now a strong case for incorporating the diagnostic and therapeutic methods outlined in the following chapters into comprehensive schemes for the prevention of osteoporosis, without further delay. But that case must rest, for the present, on the desirability of reducing fractures, disabilities and avoidable deaths, with their attendant suffering and social burdens, rather than any early savings in costs.

Bibliographical notes

Prevention of the major problems now presented by osteoporosis [e.g. Avioli L.V. (1992), Significance of osteoporosis: a growing national health care problem, *Orthop. Rev.*, **21**, 1126–9; Melton L.J. (1993), Hip fractures: a worldwide problem today and tomorrow, *Bone*, **14 suppl. 1**, S1–8] depend on *identification of those at risk, presymptomatic diagnosis, and preventive measures*, the three main headings under which the following references are grouped.

Relevant risk factors have mostly been identified in epidemiological studies [e.g. Dargent P. *et al.* (1993), Epidemiology and risk factors of osteoporosis, *Curr. Opin. Rheumatol.*, **5**, 339–45; Spector T.D. (1993), Epidemiology of the rheumatic diseases, *Curr. Opin. Rheumatol.*, **5**, 132–7; Melton L.J. *et al.* (1992), How many women have osteoporosis? *J. Bone Min. Res.*, **7**, 1005–10; Dawson-Hughes B. *et al.* (1993), Risk factors for bone loss in healthy postmenopausal women, *Osteoporos. Int.*, **3 suppl. 1**, 27–31; Peel N.F. *et al.* (1994), Distal forearm fracture as risk factor for vertebral osteoporosis, *Br. Med. J.*, **308**, 1543–4; Cummings S.R. (1993), Bone mass and bone loss in the elderly: a special case?, **38 suppl. 2**, 92–7; Cooper C. (1993), Epidemiology and public health impact of osteoporosis, *Baillières Clin. Rheumatol.*, **7**, 459–77; Cooper C. *et al.* (1993), The epidemiology of vertebral fractures. European Vertebral Osteoporosis Study Group, *Bone*, **14 suppl. 1**, S89–97; Johnston C.C. *et al.* (1993), Risk assessment: theoretical considerations, *Am. J. Med.*, **95 suppl. 5A**, 2S–5S]. Increasing attention is being paid to the risk of osteoporosis in the male [e.g. Niewoehner C.B. (1993), Osteoporosis in men. Is it more common than we think? *Postgrad. Med.*, **93**, 59–70; Seeman E. *et al.* (1983), Risk factors for spinal osteoporosis in men, *Am. J. Med.*, **75**,

977–83; Mattei J.P. *et al.* (1993), Aetiologies of male osteoporosis: identification procedures, *Clin. Rheumatol.*, **12**, 447–52].

Presymptomatic diagnosis of osteoporosis has to rely on screening, usually by means of densitometry, but only a few reports yet describe practical experience of such programs or demonstrate their value [e.g. Notelovitz M. (1993), Osteoporosis: screening, prevention, and management, *Fertil. Steril.*, **59**, 707–25; Dören M. *et al.* (1992), Identification and treatment of postmenopausal women at risk for the development of osteoporosis, *Int. J. Clin. Pharmacol. Ther. Toxicol.*, **30**, 431–3; Blumsohn A. *et al.* (1992), Prediction of bone loss in postmenopausal women, *Eur. J. Clin. Invest.*, **22**, 764–6; Lappe J.M. (1994), Bone fragility; assessment of risk and strategies for prevention, *J. Obstet. Gynecol. Neonatal Nurs.*, **23**, 260–8; Wasnich R. (1993), Bone mass measurement: prediction of risk, *Am. J. Med.*, **95 suppl. 5A**, 6S–10S]. The cost-effectiveness of screening has yet to be demonstrated [e.g. Torgerson D.J. *et al.* (1993), Osteoporosis prevention through screening: will it be cost effective?, *Baillieres Clin. Rheumatol.*, **7**, 603–22].

The cost-effectiveness of long-term preventive therapy in those identified as being at high risk also remains to be demonstrated conclusively, although evidence is accumulating [e.g. Ambrus J.L. *et al.* (1992), Prevention and treatment of osteoporosis. One of the most frequent disorders in American women: a review, *J. Med.*, **23**, 369–88; Palferman T.G. (1993), That oestrogen replacement for osteoporosis prevention should no longer be a bone of contention, *Ann. Rheum. Dis.*, **52**, 74–80; Ellerington M.C. *et al.* (1992), Prevention of osteoporosis; current recommendations, *Drugs Aging*, **2**, 508–17; Scott J.C. *et al.* (1993), Prevention of osteoporosis, *Bull. Rheum. Dis.*, **42**, 4–6; Meunier P.J. (1993), Prevention of hip fractures, *Am. J. Med.*, **95 suppl. 5A**, 75S–78S].

Chapter 5:
Early diagnosis

IF IN DOUBT, INVESTIGATE

Early diagnosis of accelerated bone loss is vital, but still uncommon. It is vital because osteoporosis can be treated preventively but not cured; lost bone can never be wholly recouped. It remains uncommon, despite increasing recognition of the disorder and greatly improved methods of investigation, because insidious changes deep in the bones draw little if any attention to themselves. No early symptoms or signs alert patient or doctor to the need for investigation. Few postmenopausal women and fewer still from other high-risk groups are yet having their bone density measured at any stage – let alone early. Hence the injunction that heads this chapter. *If in doubt, investigate.*

There is no other way to be sure what is happening to the bones of people who appear to be healthy but may already be losing bone at an accelerated rate if they belong to one or more of the high-risk groups. The earlier they are identified as being at risk and checked individually for bone loss, the sooner preventive therapy can be started. And the sooner it is started, the greater its preventive effect should be. But that is only the beginning. To be fully effective, preventive therapy also needs to be sustained – which means that its efficacy should be checked both during treatment and after withdrawal, by reinvestigating the patient's bone density. Bone is not only easy to lose and hard to recoup but easy to lose again, as symptomlessly as before.

PROPHYLACTIC WISHFUL THINKING

Growing public and medical awareness of osteoporosis has done surprisingly little to encourage large-scale screening or earlier investigation. Rather more emphasis has been placed on prophylactic measures like HRT, calcium and exercise. The latter are of course universal needs, but it does not follow that they are capable of preventing high rates of bone loss or that they will be taken consistently by those most at risk. HRT is certainly a more effective preventive measure in estrogen-deficient women – but some are at much higher risk of developing osteoporosis than others, and not all respond equally well. Yet HRT is often discussed as though it were a panacea from which postmenopausal bones are so sure to benefit that it is not necessary either to establish the individual's need for estrogen replacement, or to check the response. This is wishful thinking of a kind hitherto associated with patent medicines and quack remedies, not reputable medical prescribing.

Where initial screening, investigation and long-term follow-up should go hand-in-hand with preventive therapy of a potentially serious chronic disease like osteoporosis, some HRT is being prescribed for the purpose in an investigative vacuum. Doctor and patient are then taking too much on trust. Yet only a minority of the small proportion of postmenopausal women currently taking long-term HRT have their bone density checked beforehand and then regularly monitored to ensure that preventable bone loss is actually being prevented. Fewer still are followed up to check how severely bone loss recurs after withdrawal of HRT, as it inevitably will. Some of the many women who stop taking HRT prematurely must be at much greater risk than others, but which? Without measuring their bone density it is impossible to tell. Even those who persist for 10 years or more will start to lose bone again – silently and at an unpredictable rate – soon after HRT is discontinued. Unless their bone density continues to be monitored, those who need further preventive therapy to stem accelerated losses are most unlikely to receive it.

Without proper initial investigation, followed by monitoring of the bone density during and after a period of preventive therapy,

neither the postmenopausal patient taking HRT or other drugs nor the doctor prescribing them can possibly know where they are. Was she at high or low risk of osteoporosis in the first place? If high, have any other preventable factors contributed to her bone loss? How effective has HRT been in arresting it? Is the dose high enough? Has she been taking it regularly? Or have side-effects, or fear of them (with breast cancer often uppermost in the patient's mind) led her to abandon treatment or reduce the dose? If so, did she tell the doctor? How long does she need to continue taking HRT – or other forms of preventive therapy – for the sake of her bones? When, if ever, can all treatment be stopped without its benefits being lost within a few years? Last, but by no means least, how long should bone monitoring be continued – with or without preventive therapy – to minimize the fracture risk when it is greatest and its consequences most serious, in old age? If such questions are hard to answer for postmenopausal women on HRT, they are often more difficult in women or men requiring preventive therapy for other reasons. Without repeated measurement of the bone density they can only be answered in general terms, not necessarily relevant to a particular patient's needs.

INDIVIDUAL PATIENT CARE – BLIND OR MONITORED

The value of HRT, bisphosphonates and the other forms of preventive therapy discussed in the next chapter has been firmly established in controlled clinical trials. But this does not mean that their blind adoption in standardized dosage, perhaps taken erratically or for inadequate periods, without densitometry to monitor the response, can be relied upon to prevent bone loss or treat osteoporosis in the individual patient. Not only the peak bone mass and the subsequent rate of loss, but also the response to preventive therapy, are far too unpredictable for that.

'Blind' prescribing for more familiar conditions that can be controlled but not cured by long-term preventive therapy is open to similar objections. Nobody expects hypertension to be diagnosed without taking the blood pressure – or the dosage of antihypertensive

drugs to be adjusted without regularly monitoring the response (*Figure 1*). Still less would such treatment simply be withdrawn after a set period of, say, 5 or 10 years without further check-ups – as currently recommended for longer-term HRT in postmenopausal women. The blood pressure would almost always rise again, more dangerously so in some patients than others, just as bone loss rises after withdrawal of HRT or other forms of preventive therapy for osteoporosis. Measurement of the blood pressure is rightly recognized as being indispensable in controlling hypertension and thus for the prevention of stroke and other life-threatening or disabling complications. For blood pressure, in all patients at risk from osteoporosis, read bone density. Its measurement is no less vital in the long-term control of bone loss and therefore in the prevention of fractures and their life-threatening or disabling complications.

As the range of effective drug treatments for osteoporosis grows, its proper investigation and follow-up become more, not less, important. The greater the choice, the more informed the decisions to be made. There is no alternative to checking the bone density if appropriate preventive therapy, matched to individual needs, is to reach the majority of those at high risk early enough – and to be given in adequate dosage for long enough – to sustain an optimal response, extending into old age. The average postmenopausal woman is unwit-

Figure 1
'Nobody expects hypertension to be diagnosed without taking the blood pressure – or the dosage of antihypertensive drugs to be adjusted without regularly monitoring the response … For blood pressure, in all patients at risk from osteoporosis, read bone density.' Without densitometry, it is impossible to be sure who needs preventive therapy, how well it is working, or how long it should be continued

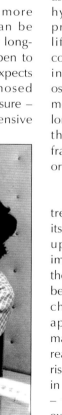

tingly caught up in a 30-years' war of attrition with osteoporosis. Some younger people may be at high risk for twice as long, yet unaware of the insidious thief persistently stealing away their bones.

Bone loss is scarcely ever self-limiting. Its treatment is no brief skirmish with an acute illness which might get better by itself or be cured by a single course of drug treatment, like giving antibiotics for an infection. There are no short cuts to the diagnosis or prevention of osteoporosis. The prophylactic strategy which starts with identifying those at risk must therefore continue with early investigation and long-term follow-up. The moral is clear, and worth reiterating. If in doubt, investigate – at any stage of suspected or established osteo-porosis, treated or untreated, in young or old. Early diagnosis must be best, but it is never too late to make a start.

DIAGNOSTIC DIFFICULTIES

Until the advent of modern methods of investigation, during the last 20 years or so, there was no reliable non-invasive technique for detecting bone loss or diagnosing osteoporosis, early or late. Neither the bone density nor the rate of loss could be accurately measured. The diagnosis was usually made late – if at all – since it had to rely quite heavily on X-ray changes and/or pathological examination of bone specimens obtained by surgical biopsy, or even postmortem.

Ordinary X-rays can only provide qualitative evidence of osteoporotic changes, not always reliably, and only when they are already quite advanced. Softening of the X-ray shadow cast by bone, suggestive of low density, can be mimicked in normal bone by the 'softness' of the exposure. Equally, osteoporotic bone loss may be masked by variations in X-ray technique. Nevertheless, some specific signs of more advanced osteoporosis should be recognizable on ordinary X-rays, notably thinning of cortical bone (*Figure 2*), the characteristic loss of horizontal

Figure 2
Ordinary X-rays often reveal signs suggestive of osteoporosis but cannot provide a measure of its severity. The Colles fracture of the forearm bones reproduced earlier (a) could easily distract attention from the cortical thinning and widened medullary canal in this 73-year-old woman. They only become obvious when compared with those of a young woman (b), though differences in X-ray exposure often confuse the issue

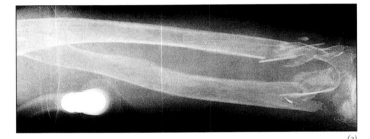

(a)

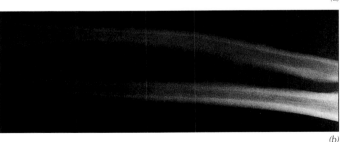

(b)

trabeculae and thickening of some vertical ones in the vertebral bodies (shown in *Figure 9*, page 48), and the rarefaction typically seen in Ward's triangle and other critical parts of the femoral neck (see *Figure 6*, page 46). But the ease, or otherwise, with which they can be detected also depends on many variables. Quite apart from the mineral density of the bone itself, these include: the duration and intensity of the X-ray exposure, the distance between the X-ray tube and the film, and the speed and contrast of its emulsion, as well as the patient's position, the size and thickness of her or his bones, and the depth of the surrounding soft tissues. The variability of each of these factors, which combine to influence the X-ray image, makes it quite impossible to measure the severity of bone loss from the depth of the images on what is, in essence, a shadowgraph (on which bones appear white only because X-ray films are negatives). All are taken under non-standardized conditions, most at short notice to reveal a fracture, or check its healing, not to identify the finer features of the bone in question, still less to measure its density.

Investigation of osteoporosis calls for measurements precise enough to detect changes in the density of trabecular bone down to as little as 1–2% of its mineral content. That cannot be achieved by examining an analogue representation of bone like an X-ray, however high its quality, even if it were scanned to digitalize the soft data its shadows represent. Accurate measurement demands hard data obtained under the rigorously standardised conditions provided by the modern methods of densitometry described later in this chapter. The first attempts to obtain standardized measurements by means of conventional radiography were only moderately successful. The best known of them, the metacarpal index, was – and still is – cheap and easy to perform using ordinary X-ray apparatus. Although much less informative and precise than modern methods, it should still be of value where special densitometry equipment is not yet available.

METACARPAL INDEX

Introduced in the 1960s as the first objective test for osteoporotic bone loss, the metacarpal index obviated assessment of the depth of X-ray 'shadow' cast by bone. Instead, the thickness of the cortex in the shaft of a metacarpal bone in the hand (or any other long bone) could be simply related to the overall diameter of its shaft at the same point (*Figure 3*). Allowance was thus automatically made for the size and strength of the individual's hand bones. The second metacarpal was usually employed for the purpose, though applying the same technique to three metacarpals (the second to fourth) in both hands has been shown to increase the reliability of the test. The necessary measurements were easy to make on an ordinary X-ray film. Little influenced by X-ray exposure or speed of emulsion, or by the small

Figure 3
Method of obtaining the metacarpal index, by relating the combined cortical thickness (AB + CD) to overall diameter (XY), usually in the mid-shaft of the second metacarpal. The cortex should represent at least half the total diameter of the shaft in young adults, to give a metacarpal index of $^1/_2$ or more. An index below $^1/_2$ is indicative of cortical bone loss. The method has been superseded by densitometry, which gives more accurate and relevant measurements of trabecular bone loss from fracture-prone sites – in the forearm, spine and hip

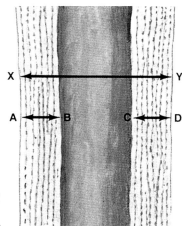

amount of soft tissue in the hand, they gave an unprecedentedly accurate and objective measure of cortical thinning, with an error well under 5%. The method nevertheless suffered from serious disadvantages.

The metacarpal index could only provide limited information about the relative thickness of cortical bone at an unimportant site, not particularly prone to fracture. The results were poorly reproducible, mainly because both cortical thickness and shaft diameter are altered by quite small differences in position, and because their shadows are magnified if the X-ray tube is brought closer to the film on which the patient's hand is resting. More seriously, because the metacarpal index measures cortical bone, it cannot tell clinicians what they most need to know: the degree of *trabecular* bone loss from the forearm, vertebral bodies, and neck of femur. At none of these sites can the metacarpal index predict the risk of fracture closely enough to be of much clinical value. This may be partly because the risk differs from one vulnerable site to another, as well as with the patient's age and other factors, but mainly because cortical bone loss normally occurs later than trabecular and is less severe. The metacarpal index is therefore of little value as an early warning sign of trabecular loss. It nevertheless ranked as an undoubted advance for a decade or more before it was superseded by single-photon absorptiometry (SPA), the first type of densitometry.

CALCIUM BALANCE

Other investigations available in the past contributed little to the diagnosis of osteoporosis. Calcium balance studies needed several days' admission to hospital, were too costly and cumbersome for routine use, and proved to be of limited value because they could only measure the comings and goings of calcium for the body as a whole. This would reveal whether a patient was in negative calcium balance – but not the reasons why, which might even include bedrest in hospital for the test to be performed! Establishing that a patient is in negative balance shows only that the bones are being drained of calcium, since they constitute the body's main reserve. It gives no information about which bones are losing mineral, how fast, or – crucially – how much remains at the sites most prone to fracture.

BONE BIOPSY

Surgical biopsy was, and still is, open to objections of a rather different nature. It gives a uniquely accurate picture of the structure and composition of the specimen examined – almost invariably trabecular bone taken from the iliac crest, because of its accessibility (*Figure 4*). This invasive, painful procedure reveals the detailed structure of bone, the exact proportions and composition of its collagen matrix and mineralization, the number and appearance of the cells and the frequency of remodelling sites. While all such

Figure 4
Bone biopsy gives 'a uniquely accurate picture of the structure and composition of the specimen obtained – almost invariably trabecular bone taken from the iliac crest, because of its availability'. It can also be used to measure new bone formation (see *Figure 15* on page 99). But bone biopsy has serious drawbacks: it is invasive, gives no reliable guide to loss of trabecular bone from the fracture-prone forearm bones, vertebral bodies or femoral neck, and cannot be readily repeated to monitor or follow-up treatment

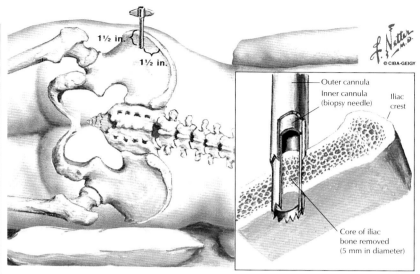

Undecalcified sections of iliac crest bone

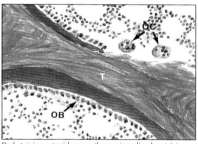

Red-staining osteoid seams (hypomineralized matrix) lined with osteoblasts (OB). Osteoclasts (OC) in resorption bays (Masson's trichrome)

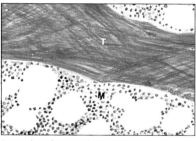

Section shows few osteoid seams, osteoblasts, or osteoclasts, indicating little bone formation or resorption
T = trabecular bone; **M** = marrow

information can be of great value in osteoporosis research, and sometimes for differential diagnosis, its clinical relevance is limited. The non-weight-bearing crest of the ilium differs radically in its trabecular structure (see *Figure 11*, page 26) from that of the well-stressed bones most liable to fracture – the distal radius and ulna, the vertebral bodies, and the neck of the femur – none of which is readily accessible for biopsy. Changes observed in the iliac crest may or may not be representative. In any case, no single biopsy could

provide a valid guide to the degree of bone loss at each of these vulnerable sites, because it differs in its timing and severity, not only from one site to another, but in each sex, and between individual patients.

Although still occasionally required in clinical practice, bone biopsies have never been widely employed in the investigation of osteoporosis – and seldom before the consequences of bone loss were painfully obvious. The surgical procedure makes biopsy wholly unsuitable for routine use as a screening test, and it could not be repeated often enough for monitoring the course of osteoporosis or its response to treatment. It can therefore contribute little to early diagnosis or follow-up. That may not have mattered greatly when little could be done to prevent or treat what was, until 20 years ago, still a little-known disease, low on the list of medical priorities. It is harder to accept the continuing failure to give higher priority to the investigation of osteoporosis and monitoring of its treatment now that the need is better understood and the necessary facilities already exist.

MISSED DIAGNOSTIC OPPORTUNITIES

Since many of the technical obstacles which precluded early diagnosis and treatment in the past have been overcome, osteoporosis could be brought under very much better control – not only in individual patients but in the population as a whole. Several non-invasive forms of densitometry can now measure the bone density and monitor the effects of treatment with unprecedented accuracy. The development of several different forms of drug treatment and demonstration of their efficacy in controlling bone loss removed the last technical hindrances to the early diagnosis, preventive therapy, and long-term follow-up of osteoporosis. Yet other hindrances remain – in the limited availability of special equipment, in the cost and possible side-effects of long-term preventive

therapy, and perhaps most of all in the minds of the many doctors and patients who still seem to be insufficiently aware of the threat that undiagnosed bone loss poses to life and wellbeing to want to do anything to prevent it.

Compelling evidence of what could now be done has been coming from a rising flood of controlled clinical trials and other research studies for over a decade. Yet the opportunity to put these lessons to large-scale use among the population as a whole is still being missed. The necessary diagnostic tests are not being carried out soon enough in sufficiently large numbers to have any appreciable impact on national statistics – though television 'advertising' of densitometry should help to remedy that, at least among postmenopausal women. It is also bound to stimulate the installation of more diagnostic equipment to meet the anticipated demand.

Largely for want of early investigation, preventive therapy is not yet being given widely enough to reduce the prime indicator of our failure to combat osteoporosis: the continuing growth in fractures as people live longer, more sedentary lives. Both in numbers and in the severity of the resulting disabilities, that growth must still be outstripping the benefits slowly accruing from advances in diagnosis and preventive therapy.

In the largest high-risk group, not one middle-aged woman in a hundred has her bones screened simply because she is post-menopausal. Yet, for that reason alone, she has an approximately even chance of becoming sufficiently osteoporotic to sustain at least one fracture, quite probably in the hip, before she dies. That average risk is far from evenly spread. Recent screening studies among postmenopausal women have shown that, at any one time, about one-third have bone densities at or below the so-called fracture threshold (*Figure 5*) – the level below which bones break unduly easily. Their risk of sustaining an osteoporotic fracture is about three times the average among postmenopausal women as a whole. Approximately half of all middle-aged and elderly women escape fractures altogether, while the other half sustain more than their fair share. To some extent this must be because they are more prone to fall, but that is not necessarily beyond the scope of preventive measures. The great majority – to judge by studies of bone density in patients who have sustained two or more fractures – have unrecognized osteoporosis. And as many as 10% of elderly patients undergoing surgery for hip fractures have been found to have some degree of osteomalacia as well. Both could be prevented by earlier investigation and appropriate drug therapy.

It is not uncommon, even today, for a woman in her fifties or sixties to have had repeated limb fractures and several collapsed vertebrae, with the loss of an inch (and sometimes much more) in height before she first undergoes densitometry or other special investigations. Fracture rates differ by several times between the majority, whose bone densities are still comfortably above the fracture threshold, and this minority. The later they are investigated for osteoporosis, the greater the danger that they will already have fallen below the fracture threshold.

FRACTURE THRESHOLD – HOW USEFUL A CONCEPT?

The fracture threshold is a somewhat nebulous concept, not altogether satisfactory as an indication of risk, and different for each bone and type of fracture. In a particular bone, it is simply the mineral density (which can now be precisely measured) below which fractures become more common (a level which has never been satisfactorily defined). It nevertheless provides a useful predictor for identifying fracture-prone bones and individuals – and thus serves as an indication for preventive therapy. Despite the fact that the threshold defined in this way only reflects the mineral content of bone, which is by no means the sole determinant

Figure 5
The mineral density of trabecular bone correlates quite well with the pattern of fractures throughout life, although the so-called fracture threshold also depends on many other factors, being no more than the level below which most fractures occur. Children's bones are always more bendy than brittle, through relatively low mineralization of their collagen matrix, and therefore liable to greenstick fractures. Older bones become brittle through loss of both collagen and mineral – which varies widely between individuals as well as being more severe in women

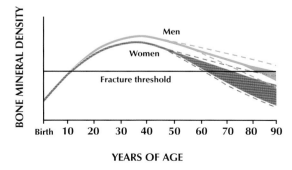

of fracture risk, it correlates quite well with the overall pattern of fractures throughout life (*Figure 6*).

No engineer could rely on such inadequate information in calculating the load a reinforced concrete beam could safely bear. It would be ridiculous to try and do so from its calcium (i.e. cement) content alone – the rough equivalent of the fracture threshold – without taking account of the quality of the concrete, the dimensions of the beam, the strength of the reinforcing bars, and the results of testing the entire beam to destruction. The true fracture threshold of a material is, after all, the minimal force required to break it. That obviously cannot be measured in human bones during life, but the threshold should ideally take account of several other relevant factors, among them likelihood of falling, the mechanism of injury, the non-mineral (collagen matrix and cellular) constituents of bone, and the force to which the fractured bone was exposed. In practice, however, none of these can be measured with any accuracy either. Hence the need to rely exclusively on the mineral content of bone as its sole property that can be measured accurately and non-invasively during life.

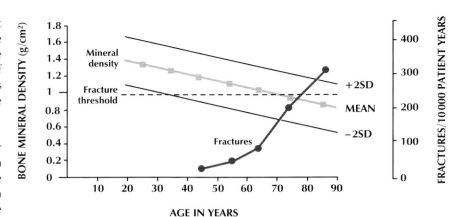

For practical purposes, the fracture threshold has been described in statistical terms as a bone density two standard deviations below the norm for people of comparable sex and age with apparently healthy bones (*Figure 6*). But such precision is a little suspect, considering the softness of the fracture data on which it has to be based. What it implies for the postmenopausal women and old people from whom most statistics have been collected is that their bone densities are already on the low side and do not have to fall very far below the norm for the risk of sustaining a fracture to rise quite sharply. This may be far from the case with physically fit young men. They can probably lose much more of their stronger bones before they even approach the fracture threshold.

SETTING NORMS

All densitometry measurements have to be set against norms, which are not universally applicable to people of the same age and sex but

Figure 6
'The fracture threshold has been described in statistical terms as a bone density two standard deviations (minus 2SD) below the norm for people of comparable age and sex…' Although the two lines do not coincide, the minus 2SD level provides measurable evidence of increased fracture risk – falling below the fracture threshold, which cannot be measured as such, by the early thirties. The mean does not do so until about 35 years later, when the fracture rate rises sharply as a result

vary with locality and ethnic origin and may also have to be modified from time to time – to take account of population movements, changes in lifestyle (eating habits, calcium intake, physical exertion, HRT, smoking, etc.) and longer-term shifts in the timetables of physical growth and sexual maturity (earlier puberty, later menopause). The norms for bone mineral in postmenopausal women and the elderly of either sex are always lower than for younger adults, because all will already have lost some bone, and an undiagnosed minority are bound to have sustained more severe losses. Consequently the norms for these high-risk groups set low standards for comparison, which decline further as age increases. The norm for a particular age and sex may

therefore fall considerably short of the optimal bone density – bringing it perilously close to the fracture threshold, especially in old age. This may help to explain why measurement of the bone density serves as a better predictor of vertebral and forearm fractures in postmenopausal women than of hip fractures in the elderly, but it is not the only reason ...

VERTEBRAL BODY FRACTURES

The vertebral bodies are exceptionally sensitive to estrogen withdrawal, not only after the natural menopause and in younger women who stop menstruating or undergo a premature or surgical menopause, but also in older ones when they stop taking estrogens in the form of HRT. In some of them, the vertebral bodies lose bone so rapidly that within 2 or 3 years they fracture more or less spontaneously. Many menopausal patients with such fractures are unaware of falls or other injuries which might have caused them. Quite often they report the sudden onset of back pain, presumably marking the moment of collapse, which may have come on for no apparent reason. This suggests that no great force was required. Weight-bearing and ordinary body movements may be sufficient to make the already-weakened trabecular bone collapse in characteristic fashion (*Figure 7*). The element of accidental injury – and thus of chance or excessive force – in the causation of these fractures must therefore be slight. In the vertebral bodies more than

Figure 7
Collapse fracture in central part of osteoporotic lumbar vertebral body (a), with dense secondary callus formation seen more clearly on X-ray (b). 'Weight-bearing and ordinary body movements may be sufficient to make the already-weakened trabecular bone collapse in characteristic fashion'. The absence of obvious accidental injury in such apparently spontaneous fractures minimizes the roles of chance and major trauma in their causation (see *Figure 8*)

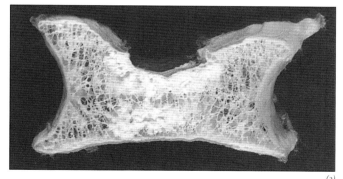

(a)

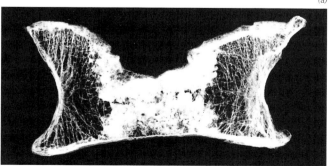

(b)

elsewhere in the skeleton, the occurrence of fractures close to threshold levels might be expected to reflect the weakness of bone – rather than external influences acting on it. This is exactly what studies have shown.

Mineral content alone allows a sharp distinction to be drawn between vertebral bodies with osteoporotic fractures and those in comparable patients which have not fractured. Loss of the collagen matrix and the radical remodelling of trabecular bone in osteoporotic vertebrae do not need to be taken into account – because the mineral content falls in line with, and thus represents, these changes. Collapse or wedging of one or more vertebral bodies occurs when the adaptive changes can no longer withstand the compressive forces imposed by everyday activities (*Figure 8*). In no other bones is the relationship between mineral density and fracture threshold so uncomplicated by trauma or chance. Together with the fact that trabecular bone is lost earlier and faster from the vertebral bodies than elsewhere, a low

mineral density in the spine, close to or below the fracture threshold, provides the clearest – and often the earliest – indication for preventive therapy.

FOREARM FRACTURES

The concept of fracture threshold, related solely to bone mineral, becomes less satisfactory in limb fractures, mainly because the leverage and impact of accidental trauma play larger but unquantifiable parts in causing them. It is impossible to be sure whether the force of a fall that caused a Colles fracture in the forearm, for instance, would have been powerful enough to break bones of greater strength. Among other factors that complicate the picture, it has been suggested that postmenopausal women are both prone to fall forwards and likely to put out an arm 'to save themselves', unaware that it may no longer be strong enough to withstand the impact. Older people, by contrast, may not be able to put out an arm quickly enough and tend to fall in more of a heap, often sustaining hip

Figure 8
'… a low mineral density in the spine, close to or below the fracture threshold, provides the clearest – and often the earliest – indication for preventive therapy.' In males with idiopathic osteoporosis (a) as well as females with postmenopausal osteoporosis (b), virtually all the vertebral fractures (black dots) fall below a mineral density of 110 mg/cm³, here determined by quantitative computer tomography (QCT – see *Figure 14*). The curves represent the normal age and sex distribution of bone mineral with 95% confidence intervals, which clearly show the earlier decline in women

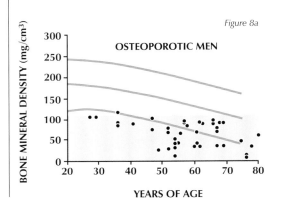

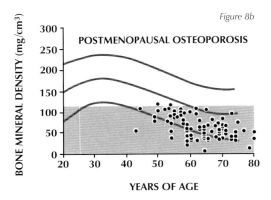

fractures. The fact that trabecular bone is lost earlier and faster than cortical may also complicate the relationship between mineral content and proneness to fracture in long bones. Having retained most of its strength, the cortical shaft may transfer much of the impact of a fall to the weaker trabecular bone which cannot withstand it. Although accidental injury plays an obvious part in causing forearm fractures, the contributions of bone loss, trauma, chance, reaction time and anatomical design should not be ignored, though none of them can be quantified. Compared with the vertebral bodies, a low fracture threshold in the forearm, based solely on mineral density, therefore provides a somewhat less clear-cut guide to the need for preventive therapy. In the hip, its value is even more questionable.

HIP FRACTURES

Determination of bone mineral in the aging femoral neck bears an uncertain relationship to the risk of hip fracture in old age and to the need for preventive therapy. Clearly, there must be a close relationship between the physical strength of the femoral neck and the force required to break it, but comparisons in old people who have and have not sustained this most disabling and life-threatening of fractures reveal little more than a trend for the mineral density to be slightly lower in the former and higher in the latter, with no sharp distinction between them.

Just where a reliable method for determining the fracture threshold is needed most, as an indicator of individual risk, measurement of the mineral density fails to provide it. Possible explanations take two main forms. Some focus on the greater risk of old people falling and of their bones taking the full impact of trauma that would often be mitigated by the quicker reflexes and stronger muscles of the young. Other explanations are based on the near-universal loss of bone from the aging femoral neck. Trabecular thinning and low bone density in critical areas like Ward's triangle (see *Figure 6*, page 46) are virtually the norm by the time women reach their seventies and eighties, having set in as much as 30–40 years earlier. The loss of bone density in men is similar, though typically running 5–10 years later, and consequently less severe at any particular age.

It needs no great medical insight to appreciate that hip fractures get progressively commoner in old age for both reasons – not only because falls become more frequent and traumatic but also because the femoral neck becomes weaker and therefore breaks more easily. The difficulty in distinguishing old people at high risk arises from there being few at low risk. There is, therefore, little scope for densitometry to single out old people of either sex as being particularly prone to hip fracture. Moreover, the measurable decline in the mineral density of old bones may be accompanied by as yet undetectable deterioration in their quality, which could well be associated with the age-related decline in osteocytes. And the femoral neck would always be more vulnerable to any consequent loss of strength than other weight-bearing bones because of the shearing forces resulting from its angular shape.

Irrespective of the reasons for femoral neck fractures rising progressively with age, the simple fact that the bone mineral density does not provide a clear measure of the risk in those who are already old has obvious clinical implications. To have any appreciable preventive value, densitometry of the hip should be performed earlier – preferably in the fifties or sixties, not in old age when much bone has already been lost and the threat of fracture is imminent. In short, we should not play at brinkmanship with the fracture threshold, least of all in the hip. It ought to be treated with the respect that a sailor pays to a rocky lee shore in stormy weather. In other words, it is best kept well clear of in old age, to avert the risk of femoral shipwreck.

The opportunity to maintain a safety margin over and above the fracture threshold is currently being missed, and not only in the femoral neck. Investigations are done too late, if at all. Silent bone loss simply continues, unsuspected by those unknowingly at risk, undiagnosed by their doctors and therefore uncontrolled. *If* – sadly, one cannot say *when* – tests are belatedly done

for osteoporosis, the fracture threshold may already have been breached. Even if it is only drawing too close for comfort, the best opportunity for preventive therapy will long since have been lost.

REVEALING FACTS – AND A FEW FALLACIES

The investigations of greatest value for diagnosing osteoporosis and monitoring the response to preventive therapy are of two main types, of which the first is by far the most important at present:

Densitometry, which employs various scanning techniques to measure the mineral content (or so-called 'density') of bone, and

Biochemical tests of bone turnover, based on measurement, in the blood or urine, of various compounds which are actively concerned in, or metabolic products of, the twin processes of bone resorption and/or new bone formation.

The sophisticated techniques now available in both fields represent successive advances, made over the past 20 years or more, which are still continuing and promise further improvements in the future. They already give the doctor unprecedentedly accurate and reliable information about the state of the bones and current trends in their turnover by non-invasive methods, which are both repeatable when necessary and acceptable to patients. All, nonetheless, have their limitations.

ESTIMATING BONE MASS AND RATES OF LOSS

Neither the peak bone mass nor the rate of bone loss can be measured as such, invaluable though they are as twin concepts governing the severity of all osteoporosis. The peak bone mass is a movable feast occurring at various times in different bones, even in different parts of the same bone, during the first decade or more of adult life. No attempt is made to measure it in clinical practice. Nor is enough yet known from research studies about when the bone mass peaks, in which bones, or for how long, for any norms to have been established. It should be practicable to settle on a standardized densitometry procedure for its measurement in specified bones at a certain age, perhaps between the ages of 25 and 30. International agreement on such a procedure would not only facilitate research but ultimately contribute to individual patient care.

In girls and others predictably at long-term risk, the peak bone mass, measured by a standardized screening procedure, could be used as an individual baseline for the assessment of later densitometry findings, particularly after the menopause. But that is not yet possible. At present, the patient's own peak bone mass is never available as a basis for comparison. Densitometry readings, therefore,

have to be set against local averages for people of the same age and sex and/or their hypothetical peak bone mass. There are no firm baseline data to go on except the first bone density values obtained in a particular patient, usually after the menopause when an unknown quantity of bone has already been lost.

The rate of bone loss also has to be estimated. In the short term (days or weeks), this can be done by measuring chemical markers of bone resorption, set against those for new bone formation – though this only allows some limited conclusions to be drawn about the overall balance between them in the skeleton as a whole. Like calcium balance studies, it provides no specific measurements of trabecular bone loss at vulnerable sites, and has yet to find an established place in clinical practice. In the rather longer term (months or years), bone loss can be accurately determined at sites of interest by repeating densitometry at intervals and comparing the results with earlier findings.

WHAT TESTS DO AND DO NOT REVEAL

Whereas densitometry focuses exclusively on deficiency of bone mineral, the biochemical tests described at the end of this chapter give more information about the turnover of collagen matrix reflecting the processes of its resorption and synthesis as well as its subsequent mineralization. But no non-invasive tests reveal anything about the numbers or functioning of the osteocytes, on which bone quality may depend in old age, or about the quantity or normality of the collagen matrix. Densitometry can do no more than show, by implication, that there must be enough matrix to carry the quantity of mineral demonstrated. Low mineral readings, which are usually accepted as evidence of osteoporosis, could equally well mean that the matrix is under-mineralized. Indeed, osteomalacia would almost certainly have been the main cause of low mineral density in western countries until early in the present century. Adults who lack vitamin D are no less vulnerable to it today – as shown by the recent demonstration of osteomalacia coexisting with osteoporosis in elderly patients undergoing hip surgery. Low densitometry readings do not represent a diagnosis of osteoporosis or necessarily enable it to be distinguished from osteomalacia.

There are some situations in which bone mineral of little or no structural merit could give misleadingly high densitometry readings. Exostoses and other bony prominences, including the dense ridges which develop around joint margins, which are common in the middle-aged and elderly age groups prone to osteoporosis, particularly affecting those with osteoarthritis, can considerably add to the apparent mineral content of bone without increasing its strength commensurately. In some forms of

densitometry they have to be excluded, so far as possible, by outlining the vertebral bodies and hip bones. It is less easy to exclude the effect of fluoride, however, whether prescribed for osteoporosis or naturally present in the water supply at high concentrations (several times higher than those added to strengthen the teeth). Excessive fluoride has the effect of stimulating the formation of poorly organized bone with a physical strength lower than its mineral content suggests.

For all these limitations, which must always be considered in assessing the significance of densitometry, it provides the best clinical measure of bone strength available at present. The fact that it can be performed non-invasively by a variety of methods, with increasing speed and accuracy, makes it the most practical means of assessing both the need for, and the response to, preventive therapy.

DENSITOMETRY – IN PRINCIPLE AND PRACTICE

Four main types of densitometry, each measuring the mineral density by a different technique, are currently in clinical use:

1) Single-photon absorptiometry (SPA),

2) Dual-photon absorptiometry (DPA),

3) Dual-energy X-ray absorptiometry (DXA), and

4) Quantitative computer tomography (QCT).

In addition, ultrasonography (US) and nuclear magnetic resonance (NMR) can be adapted to measure bone mineral, and these methods may be further developed in the future. All these methods employ scanning mechanisms which rely on the same basic principle of absorptiometry, i.e. measurement of the energy differentially absorbed from a photon, X-ray, or ultrasonic beam as it passes through different parts of the body. Bone absorbs much more than other tissues because of, and in proportion to, its mineral content. In effect, scanning measures the density of the 'shadow' cast by bone, and this enables its mineral content to be calculated, often at the cost of detail. The earlier scanning systems in particular showed a rather crude outline of the bones examined and little or nothing of their internal structure. Loss of trabecular and cortical bone may then be impossible to distinguish in areas like the vertebral bodies where they coexist. These problems are being overcome by DXA and QCT, and the high accuracy with which densitometry can measure the mineral content of bone is still being improved. All the methods in current use are non-invasive, none exposes the patient to any significant hazard or inconvenience – and costs are tending to fall as scan times are reduced.

Single-photon absorptiometry (SPA)

Modern densitometry began in the 1970s with introduction of the first scanning technique, single-photon absorptiometry, which is still in

Figure 9
Single-photon absorptiometry (SPA), the first reliable method of densitometry, is still useful for measuring the mineral content of smaller long bones, typically the radius. The method is simple, quick, non-invasive, and useful as a screening test, but unsuitable for densitometry of the hip or spine. The water-bath, here shown as a cuff, standardizes the variable thickness of soft tissues, which would otherwise distort the results

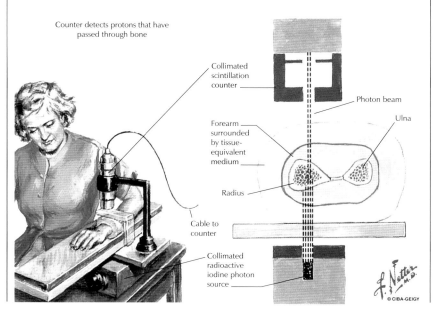

Counter detects protons that have passed through bone

Collimated scintillation counter

Photon beam

Ulna

Forearm surrounded by tissue-equivalent medium

Radius

Cable to counter

Collimated radioactive iodine photon source

© CIBA-GEIGY

quite widespread use. The photons employed are emitted from a radio-isotope, usually [125]iodine, in a single collimated beam, which scans the area to be investigated in parallel lines, building up a two-dimensional image via a scintillation counter, much as a television picture is formed, though much less rapidly. This digitalized scan accurately reflects the relatively high degree of photon absorption by bone (compared with soft tissue), which is directly proportional to its mineral content. The latter is normally expressed as grams per centimeter of linear scan.

The patient undergoing SPA only has to sit quietly with the forearm – or occasionally the lower leg – in a water bath for some minutes (*Figure 9*). The equipment is relatively simple and inexpensive, which enabled it to become quite widely available without much delay. Exposure to radiation is low enough for the test to be repeated when necessary. The bone mineral measurements are accurate (to within less than 2%) and highly reproducible on successive examinations or between different centers. Against these considerable advantages over any previous form of investigation for osteoporosis, the only appreciable drawbacks of SPA arise from its limited applications and sensitivity to interference by soft tissues, especially fat. The waterbath minimizes this by creating a uniform thickness of soft-tissue and liquid (of similar density) combined, which is most easily arranged for the forearm bones. Reliable information can be obtained about the mineral content of their cortical (mid-shaft) and trabecular (distal radius) components, depending on the level at which the test is carried out (*Figure 10*). For the first time, SPA

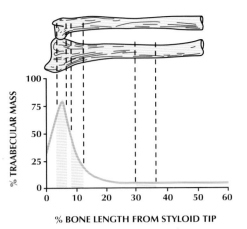

Figure 10
The distribution of trabecular bone in the radius, showing how densitometry can be used at different levels to measure the mineral content of predominantly cortical or trabecular bone. As in all long bones, the mid-shaft of the radius is well over 90% cortical bone, whereas trabecular bone fills 80% of the distal expansion at its broadest point

Figure 11
Dual-photon absorptiometry (DPA) extended photon absorption to larger bones in the hip region and spine, deeper in the body. Although DPA can provide accurate measurements, the method is slow, definition of the scans is poor (as shown here), not enabling trabecular bone to be distinguished from cortical in the hip or spine. DPA has now been largely superseded by the more versatile X-ray absorptiometry based on the same dual-energy principle (see *Figures 12 and 13*)

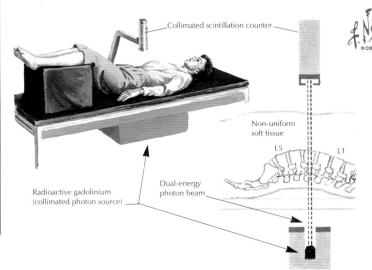

Collimated scintillation counter

Non-uniform soft tissue

Radioactive gadolinium (collimated photon source)

Dual-energy photon beam

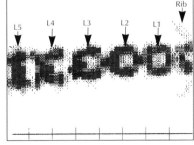

Bone mineral content determined by measuring attenuation of photons passing through body tissues. Dual energy source separates mineral mass from soft tissue mass, which is abundant and non-uniform in lumbar region. Density of vertebrae determined from computerized printout

made it possible to measure the mineral density of trabecular and cortical bone with great accuracy, and thus to assess their proneness to fracture.

Dual-photon absorptiometry (DPA)

Densitometry could only be extended to the spine and the hip region by the development of a technique less subject to soft-tissue interference. This need was initially fulfilled by dual-photon absorptiometry, which employs a radio-isotope (^{153}gadolinium) that emits photon beams at two distinct energy levels (44 and 100 keV). The differential between them enables interference from fat and other soft tissues to be effectively eliminated. Bone mineral can thus be measured with considerable accuracy, deep within the body, using acceptably low levels of radiation (*Figure 11*). Dual-photon absorptiometry has now been largely superseded by faster methods giving more information with even lower exposure to radiation. The two newer methods returned to X-rays, in digitalized rather than analogue form, the more important of them employing a modification of the dual-energy principle.

Dual-energy X-ray absorptiometry (DXA)

The use of dual-energy X-rays in place of a dual-photon emitting radio-isotope reduces the radiation exposure to negligible levels well within the most stringent safety limits, and allows the investigation to be performed much more rapidly, thus reducing costs. For most purposes, DXA is now the investigation of choice, which has set new standards in the diagnosis of osteoporosis. The radiation required is so low that patients can be re-investigated as often as necessary and the operator needs no special protection. DXA can be used to examine the vertebral bodies and hip region, as well as the forearm bones, with unprecedented speed and accuracy (*Figures 12 and 13*). The time needed for each scan has already fallen to just a few minutes, without loss of accuracy, and promises to fall to no

Figure 12
Dual-energy X-ray absorptiometry (DXA) has significant advantages over DPA in lower radiation exposure, faster screening with quicker throughput of patients, and a greater range of techniques. It is now the investigation of choice for osteoporosis, equally suitable for rapid screening, detailed evaluation, monitoring of the response to treatment, and long-term follow-up. The X-ray scanning process (a) resembles DPA but is much quicker for the patient (b) and therefore more acceptable and cheaper as well as more informative

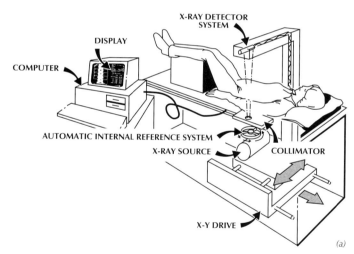

(a)

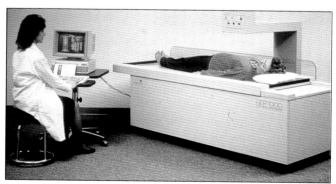

(b)

more than 10–20 seconds. For all these reasons, DXA is as well suited to screening of postmenopausal women and others at risk, and to monitoring of preventive therapy as it is to full investigation of patients with established osteoporosis. Further developments, such as lateral examination of the vertebral bodies (*Figure 13c*) and whole-body measurements (*Figure 13d*), have extended the scope of DXA, making it the most versatile and generally useful method for measuring the bone mineral. The results are accurate and easily read, allowing small changes to be reliably detected.

Quantitative computer tomography (QCT)

In contrast to photon and X-ray absorptiometry, which require dedicated equipment unsuitable for other diagnostic purposes, computer-assisted tomography is already available in most major hospitals. The CT (or CAT) scans it normally produces are cross-sections through any desired part of the body, built up by computer manipulation of data obtained by X-ray scanning (*Figure 14*). Unlike ordinary X-ray films, the resulting images represent detailed tomographic 'slices' through the body at different depths, which requires higher radiation but shows the internal organs and other soft tissues as clearly as the bone structure. But the CT scans which have so enhanced the scope of X-ray diagnosis in many fields of medicine are still analogue

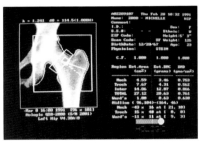

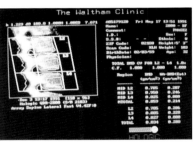

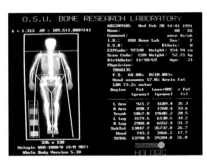

representations, built up into a picture from digitally manipulated data. To obtain measurements of bone mineral, the CT scanning data have to be quantitated and presented in numerical form. This is

Figure 13
Typical DXA visual displays with print-outs of precise bone density data, obtained on the Hologic QDR-2000.

(a) Postero-anterior scan of lumbar spine, showing the first four lumbar vertebrae outlined for measurement with the bone mineral content and density data for each

(b) Left hip with data for each of the four areas of interest scanned, including the poorly mineralized Ward's triangle

(c) Lateral scan of lumbar spine with the vertebral bodies both outlined and containing a fainter 'box' for determining the density of the central area of exclusively trabecular bone

(d) DXA can also be used for measuring total body calcium and monitoring changes in it, providing a simpler, cheaper and more informative alternative to calcium balance studies

at present a more costly type of densitometry than DXA, but it does provide more comprehensive diagnostic information.

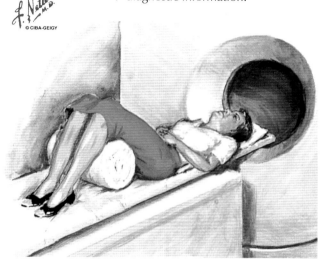

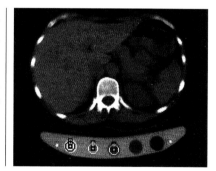

Figure 14
Quantitative computer tomography (QCT) is a specialized form of the CT scanning used for brain scans and other diagnostic purposes. It requires considerably higher X-ray exposure than DXA, but has the advantage of providing higher resolution pictures of bone and soft tissues as well as quantifying bone density. In osteoporosis, it is used mainly in research studies and sometimes for differential diagnosis

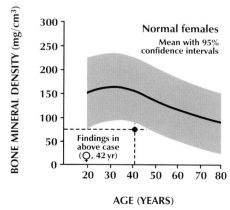

OTHER FORMS OF DENSITOMETRY

Two diagnostic imaging techniques which do not expose patients to X-rays or other forms of radiation can be adapted to investigation of osteoporosis: *ultrasonography and nuclear magnetic resonance*. The former works on an echo-sounding principle similar to that developed during the Second World War to detect enemy submarines under water. Their metal hulls produced a recognizable 'echo', compared with the surrounding water, much as bones do in contrast to soft tissues. Because cortical bone is so much more compact than trabecular bone, they can also be distinguished from one another, and there are prospects for refining the measurement of bone density by this non-hazardous and inexpensive technique. Like QCT, it could have the advantage of employing equipment already in use for other diagnostic purposes.

Although far from cheap, nuclear magnetic resonance (NMR) also has the advantages of wider investigative value and lack of radiation. It relies instead on exposing the body quite briefly to intense magnetism inside a large electromagnet and has great diagnostic potential which has scarcely begun to be applied to osteoporosis. Magnetic resonance imaging (MRI) may well find a place in the specialized investigation of osteoporosis and possibly in screening. Further technical advances could lead to wider applications in the future, possibly including investigation of metabolic activity in the bones, as forecast in the last chapter.

BIOCHEMICAL TESTS OF BONE TURNOVER

For many years after biochemical tests first started to be applied to the investigation of osteoporosis, their results were too often normal or inconclusive to be of much value in its diagnosis. That position has only changed appreciably in recent years, with the refinement of old tests and development of new ones, the most important of which are summarized in Table 1.

Serum *calcium* and *phosphorus* levels are typically within the normal range in osteoporotic patients. The only major exceptions are certain types of secondary osteoporosis – associated with parathyroid disorders, for example – and patients with bone metastases, who often have pathologically high serum calcium levels. Measurement of the serum calcium is, therefore, principally of use in excluding pathological causes of osteoporosis or other types of serious bone disease.

Serum levels of the enzyme *alkaline phosphatase* are also normal in osteoporotic patients, except in those with healing fractures, but consistently raised in patients with osteomalacia and also in patients with bone secondaries. Elevated levels in an osteoporotic patient not known to have had a recent fracture are therefore suggestive of osteomalacia and/or secondaries or undiagnosed fractures of the vertebral bodies. Testing is not now confined to the conventional *total* alkaline phosphatase levels in the serum, but can also be done for the

Table 1 Biochemical tests of bone turnover – in the body as a whole		
Test	**Result in osteoporosis**	**Diagnostic value**
Blood/serum tests		
Calcium	normal range	exclusion of parathyroid disease, bone metastases, etc.
Alkaline phosphatase (total)	normal range	exclusion of healing fractures, bone metastases, etc.
Bone-specific alkaline phosphatase	raised if osteoblast activity high	specific measure of new bone formation
Bone Gla-protein (osteocalcin)	raised by active synthesis of bone matrix	specific measure of new bone formation
Urine tests		
Hydroxyproline excretion	raised if collagen breakdown high	non-specific measure of collagen resorption
Pyridinium cross-links excretion	raised if resorption of bone collagen high	specific measure of bone resorption
Bone biopsy		
Tetracycline labelling (see *Figure 15*)	depends on activity of bone formation and mineralization	assessment of bone turnover; used mainly in research studies

bone-specific isoenzyme. This is a valuable distinction, because serum concentrations of *bone-specific alkaline phosphatase* reflect levels of activity in the osteoblasts which produce it.

Bone Gla-protein (BGP), or *osteocalcin*, is a non-collagenous component of normal bone matrix, also present in dentine. Since some spills over into the bloodstream during bone synthesis (but not from adult teeth), measurement of its serum levels by radioimmunoassay provides a useful measure of bone formation.

For a long time, there was no corresponding biochemical test giving a reliable measure of bone resorption. Urinary excretion of the collagen breakdown product *hydroxyproline* was not specific for bone collagen – and therefore of little value in view of collagen being the most plentiful tissue in the body. This has now changed with the development of highly specific tests for *pyridinium cross-links* which are found only in bone collagen. Excretion of this breakdown product provides a measure of the rate of bone resorption – in the body as a whole, of course.

Taken together, these tests not only exclude other conditions but help to confirm the presence of osteoporosis. They also make it possible to draw up a balance between resorption and new bone formation. This has the potential to show whether these remodelling processes are running at a net loss – in the body as a whole – and also enables the rate of bone turnover to be assessed. Both pieces of information may help to indicate suitable forms of preventive therapy, as noted in the next chapter. Biochemical tests can also be used, alongside densitometry, to check the course of therapy and the

degree of imbalance in remodelling activity after its withdrawal.

Where tetracycline labelling and bone biopsy have sometimes been used to assess the rate of bone turnover, and also to exclude osteomalacia (*Figure 15*), biochemical tests now seem likely to replace these methods. A biochemical profile has also been evaluated as a possible screening test for osteoporosis, among other proposed uses. With the battery of tests now available, it would be surprising if they did not come to play a more important collective part in the initial investigation and the long-term management of osteoporosis. If even more refined biochemical tests are developed in the future, as seems quite probable, they could come to sit alongside or even rival densitometry in importance. They are capable of giving much more information, perhaps more cheaply, about what is happening to bone, here and now, rather than over the preceding months and years. Treatment could then be tailored not only to the individual patient but to correct the specific imbalances in bone remodelling responsible for that particular patient's bone loss.

Figure 15
The antibiotic tetracycline binds to mineral newly laid down at remodelling sites (and can discolor children's teeth in much the same way). Three days' dosage is sufficient to stain new mineral with a thin line which fluoresces yellow. If this is repeated after 14 days, the distance between the fluorescent lines gives a measure of the rate of bone mineralization (a). Absence of tetracycline labelling denotes lack of new bone formation (b)

T = trabecular bone; **M** = marrow

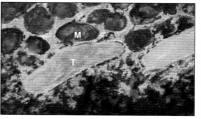

(a)

(b)

Bibliographical notes

Recent references to investigative methods are grouped under three main headings: general diagnosis, densitometry for measurement of bone mineral, and biochemical markers, mainly of bone matrix turnover.

Several papers consider diagnosis as a whole [e.g. Nordin B.E. (1994), Guidelines for bone densitometry, *Med. J. Aust.*, **160**, 517–20; Jergas M. *et al.* (1993), Current methods and recent advances in the diagnosis of osteoporosis, *Arthritis Rheum.*, **36**, 1649–62; Mitlak B.H. *et al.* (1993), Diagnosis and treatment of osteoporosis, *Annu. Rev. Med.*, **44**, 265–77; Sambrook P. *et al.* (1993), Diagnosis and treatment of osteoporosis, *Curr. Opin. Rheumatol.*, **5**, 346–50].

Densitometry methods have been critically reviewed by several leading authorities [e.g. Delmas P.D. (1993), Bone mass measurement: how, where, when and why? *Int. J. Fertil Menopausal Stud.*, **38 suppl. 2**, 70–6; Grampp S. *et al.* (1993), Radiologic diagnosis of osteoporosis. Current methods and objectives, *Radiol. Clin. North Am.*, **31**, 1133–45; Greenfield M.A. (1992), Current status of physical measurements of the skeleton, *Med. Physics*, **19**, 1349–57]. More specialized studies have addressed particular problems [e.g. Flynn M.J. et al. (1993), The assessment of vertebral bone macroarchitecture with X-ray computed tomography, *Calcif. Tissue Int.*, **53 suppl. 1**, S170–5; Wehrli F.W. *et al.* (1993), Potential role of nuclear magnetic resonance for the evaluation of trabecular bone quality, *Calci. Tissue Int.*, **53 suppl. 1**, S162–9], while others have challenged the value of densitometry [e.g. Ribot C. *et al.* (1993), Is absorptiometry useful? (French, editorial), *Rev. Rheum Ed. Fr.*, **60**, 321–3; Ott S.M. (1993), When bone mass fails to predict bone failure, *Calcif. Tissue Int.*, **53 suppl. 1**, 7–13].

More reports are now being devoted to biochemical markers, as they become more numerous and extend their diagnostic value [e.g. Ohishi T. *et al.* (1994), Urinary bone resorption markers in patients with metabolic bone disorders, *Bone*, **15**, 15–20; Delmas P.D. (1993), Biochemical markers of bone turnover. I. Theoretical considerations and clinical use in osteoporosis, *Am. J. Med.*, **95 suppl. 5A**, 11S–16S; Riis B.J. (1993), Biochemical markers of bone turnover. II. Diagnosis, prophylaxis and treatment of osteoporosis, *Am. J. Med.*, **95 suppl. 5A**, 17S–21S; Delmas P.D. (1993), Biochemical markers of bone turnover, *J. Bone Min. Res.*, **8 suppl. 2**, S549–55; Reid, D.M. (1993), Measurement of bone turnover and clinical investigation of osteoporosis; relevance to asthma and corticosteroid therapy, *Respir. Med.*, **87 suppl. A**, 9–14].

Chapter 6:
Preventive therapy

TAILORING TREATMENT TO INDIVIDUAL NEEDS

Preventive therapy has the power to revolutionize the management of osteoporosis – within limits. Although preventive, it cannot act like a dose or two of vaccine to give lifelong protection from bone loss. Although therapeutic, it offers no quick or lasting cure of the kind commonly produced by a short course of antibiotics and now expected of many modern drugs. There are, as yet, no such short cuts to the prevention or treatment of osteoporosis. Its preventive therapy must, therefore, be seen in the lifelong context of bone's natural history (Table 1). None of the drugs

developed in recent years provides an effective substitute for building up the bone mass in youth or for the conditions required to maintain it thereafter. Taken as a whole, these drugs are simply the most effective means yet found for combatting excessive bone loss – at any age – when the body fails to do so.

All osteoporosis, irrespective of age or sex, arises from failure of the body's feedback control mechanisms to bring bone remodelling into balance. That is the gap in nature's providence which preventive therapy has to fill – either by curbing unduly high rates of resorption, or by generating new bone fast enough to keep pace. The circumstances in

Table 1 Preventive therapy in context: its place in the natural history of bone		
Phase of life/ circumstances	**Aims**	**Prophylactic measures**
Infancy Childhood Adolescence	build up strong bones (especially in girls)	calcium, vitamin D, exercise, etc. *Avoid adverse factors:* amenorrhea, excessive slimness, smoking, etc.
Early adulthood	attain optimal peak bone mass	continue above
Throughout adult life	maintain bone density	continue above
Amenorrhea Corticosteroid therapy Surgical menopause Testosterone deficiency Postmenopausal women Old of both sexes Other risk groups	identify those at high risk and curb excessive bone loss to prevent osteoporotic fractures	screen for low bone density and/or rapid bone loss **Preventive therapy: HRT, bisphosphonates, calcitonin, fluorides, anabolic steroids, etc.** *plus:* **calcium, vitamin D, exercise, and avoidance of risk factors**
Lifelong	check response	**Monitor bone density before, during and after withdrawal of treatment**

which such measures are needed arise predominantly, though by no means exclusively, in later life (*Figure 1*). Indeed, bone loss is so universal among postmenopausal women and elderly people of both sexes, and follows such characteristic patterns in each, as to represent the physiological norm. In other words, the threat that osteoporosis now poses in these major groups, constituting about a quarter of the entire population in industrialized countries, cannot be regarded as truly abnormal, despite its pathological consequences. It is far too commonplace for that. As shown earlier, the high risk of fracture to which postmenopausal women and older people are now exposed has not resulted from increased disease or exposure to adverse environmental influences but, paradoxically, from the improvements in living conditions and advances in treatment that have strikingly lengthened the average lifespan.

MAN-MADE THREATS . . .

Bone loss must have followed the menopause and accompanied aging throughout human history – in the few who survived past middle age. It now puts unprecedented numbers at risk because most people are outliving the strength of their bones. This is numerically the most important way in which human activities have inadvertently increased the need for preventive measures – which few of those at high risk yet take. Although less common, the increase in bone loss that now afflicts younger age groups is always

abnormal and therefore arguably more important. It represents a more prolonged, even a lifelong threat to the skeleton, for which the comparative youth of those at risk fails to compensate. The recent growth in osteoporosis among younger adults has also arisen from human activities, as though modern life were challenging the body, to expose the weak points in its defences. Yet when they are breached and bone loss results, it often goes unrecognized – and

consequently unchecked. Regrettably, this even happens when the challenge takes the apparently benign form of advances in treatment for other conditions.

Long-term corticosteroid therapy and premature induction of the menopause by ablation or removal of the ovaries must be the commonest causes of osteoporosis in younger adults. Both are twentieth century developments calling for preventive therapy. But the bone loss caused by these novel forms of treatment was not properly understood when they were first introduced, and could not

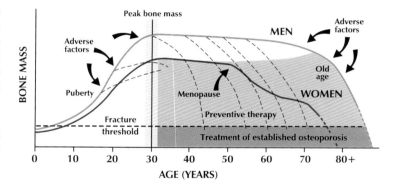

Figure 1
Indications for the prevention and treatment of osteoporosis. The need for preventive therapy to control bone loss increases as the bone mass declines, especially after the menopause and in old age (as shown by light pink shading). Prevention cannot be sharply distinguished from treatment for established osteoporosis, which becomes imperative below the notional fracture threshold (dark pink area). Despite the development of effective drugs for both purposes, most opportunities to prevent bone loss or treat osteoporosis are still missed

then have been adequately controlled. That the risk of osteoporosis too often continues to go unchecked in such patients today may be partly an unfortunate legacy from the past. Certainly, this potentially serious side-effect of well-intentioned treatments is still underestimated by many doctors prescribing them, with the result that their patients are deprived of the preventive therapy now widely available.

Human activities of less salutary kinds must bear much of the responsibility for the sinister triad of persistent amenorrhea, estrogen deficiency and bone loss, which afflicts many younger women today, often because they are abnormally thin through intensive physical exercise, obsessional dieting or falling victim to stress-related behavioral disorders like anorexia, bulimia or drug addiction. Even among otherwise healthy young women who do menstruate regularly, many must have a suboptimal bone mass partly attributable to calcium deficiency in childhood and adolescence. About one-third must also be losing bone at an enhanced rate because the effectiveness of their own estrogens is reduced by smoking. And yet another medical threat to the female skeleton is already on the horizon. A long-acting contraceptive has been developed that, in contrast to the estrogen in existing ones, which tends to strengthen the bones, will persistently lower the natural estrogen levels in women of childbearing age.

Apart from the modest beneficial effect of oral contraceptives and the development of HRT and other forms of preventive therapy, the various adverse factors that increase the risk of osteoporosis are not being counterbalanced by modern trends that protect or strengthen the bones. Quite the opposite. The hazards to which the skeleton is now exposed are commonly being exacerbated by inattention to its basic needs for adequate calcium, vitamin D, first-class protein (mainly from meat) and physical exertion in childhood, and by the decline in manual labor and milk consumption among adults. Many people, and especially young women, must now be entering adult life with a suboptimal peak bone mass. They are therefore ill-equipped to face the variety of osteoporotic challenges the modern world has in store for their bones.

... REQUIRING MAN-MADE SOLUTIONS

Why should the body possess so few built-in countermeasures to meet such challenges? Probably because most adults were of breeding age throughout the long course of human evolution. The bones of both men and women would, therefore, have been kept strong by their sex hormones, since nature always gives priority to propagation and adaptation of the species. Osteoporosis would rarely have threatened these vital processes in the past – and natural selection, being based exclusively on practical experience of the real world, never insures against hypothetical threats. Indeed it has no means of doing so. Survival of the fittest can only operate when those young enough to breed are exposed to actual hazards.

Natural selection is a harsh doctrine. It callously overlooks those who are infertile in youth or unable to propagate their kind because they are past reproductive age – unless they happen to contribute to the survival of the young. That could originally have been the evolutionary advantage of human longevity. But the modern world that has so strikingly increased the average lifespan has also made grandparents socially redundant, more of a burden on younger generations than

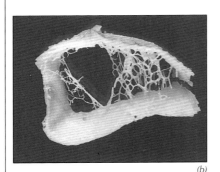

(b)

an aid to their survival. Evolution cannot, therefore, be expected to combat the ills of the infertile or the elderly. Even if it could, countless generations would be needed for human biology to adapt to the problems now posed by osteoporosis. Whether anything effective is done more promptly to protect the human skeleton from the added risks to which we now so carelessly expose it therefore depends, appropriately enough, upon our own efforts.

That more should be done to promote the strength of the growing skeleton has already been shown in earlier chapters. The emphasis here is on preventing excessive bone loss in adult life and rebuilding what has already been lost – so far as that is

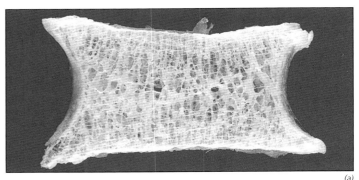

(a)

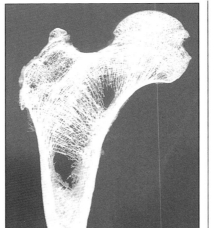

(c)

Figure 2
The main targets for preventive therapy: the three areas of osteoporotic bone most prone to fracture, shown as sections that reveal their inner weaknesses. The vertebral bodies (a) lose bone rapidly during the 2 years or so of high turnover that follow estrogen withdrawal in women, at or before the menopause. They and the distal radius (b) commonly fracture in recently menopausal women. Hip fractures, mostly through the osteoporotic neck of the femur (c), are more frequent in old people of both sexes but remain more common in women

possible – because little can yet be done to correct the fundamental causes of osteoporosis. It is seldom possible to restore natural production of the body's own sex hormones, except by encouraging an abnormally thin young woman with amenorrhea to exercise less and eat more, so that she puts on enough weight to start menstruating regularly again. There are rarely substitutes for corticosteroid treatment in the many patients who need it. Female fertility cannot be extended beyond the menopause without resort to another woman's ova, developing in a contrived hormonal milieu. And there is certainly no way to slow the aging process – despite some of the wilder claims made for the rejuvenating effects of HRT.

Table 2 The main classes of preventive therapy

Hormone replacement therapy (HRT)

For postmenopausal and amenorrheic younger women with low bone density, to prevent further loss by correcting estrogen deficiency

Conjugated equine estrogens, by mouth
Estradiol, transdermal absorption from skin patches – also tablets, subcutaneous implants, and creams (mainly for local application to vulva and vagina)
Other estrogen preparations (see *Table 3*)

Any woman with an intact uterus should also take a *progestogen* cyclically, for 10–14 days each month (see *Table 6*)

For testosterone-deficient men with low bone density to prevent further loss

Testosterone preparations – transdermal absorption from skin patches, tablets, or subcutaneous implants

Drugs other than sex hormones

For men or women with low bone density, whether deficient in sex hormones or not

Bisphosphonates, usually by mouth, can be injected
Calcitonin, by nasal inhalation or injection
Anabolic steroids, by mouth or injection
Fluoride salts, by mouth
Calcium and vitamin D supplements, especially in old age

General measures

For all children, adolescents and adults of either sex, irrespective of bone density, sex hormone status or preventive therapy

Everybody needs: Adequate calcium, vitamin D, and physical exercise

Women also need: Training in good spinal posture

Women should avoid: All adverse factors that cause amenorrhea or reduce estrogen activity: anorexia, undue thinness, excessive exercise, heroin addiction, cigarette smoking, etc.

Postmenopausal women, old people of both sexes, and the fracture-prone of any age should also: Take calcium and vitamin D supplements, and seek to minimize the risk of falls and fractures

---

Greater attention to the needs of the growing skeleton and to its maintenance throughout adult life, by means of HRT and other forms of preventive therapy, offer the only present prospects of reducing vulnerability to osteoporotic fractures (*Figure 2*) and the widespread disabilities they cause.

TYPES OF PREVENTIVE THERAPY

The various drugs available today, and the fact that they curb bone loss in different ways, mean that all types of osteoporosis can now be treated preventively at any stage, in men as well as women, whatever their age. It is no longer necessary to ask if anything *can* be done to protect those at risk. Attention is therefore shifting to more practical questions: how to identify those at risk in good time, what sort of preventive therapy is most appropriate for particular patients, how to persuade them to take it regularly, how effective it will prove, and how long it should be continued. The customary distinctions between prevention and treatment are relatively unimportant. Virtually all the drugs and general measures discussed in this chapter can serve either purpose, depending on the severity of each patient's bone loss. In practice, their prescribing may be regarded as treatment for patients with bone densities below the fracture threshold, and prevention for those above this nebulous border (*see Figure 1*). The drugs of proven value for either purpose form two main groups, both summarized in Table 2 together with a third category of general prophylactic measures, particularly important in women.

1. *Hormone replacement* is the most physiological form of prevention or treatment for osteoporosis. Estrogens in women and testosterone in men act chiefly by inhibiting the excessive bone resorption, and also by improving the poor absorption of dietary calcium, which both result from their own deficiency. Testosterone also has some direct stimulant effect on bone formation, much as it stimulates muscle development in the male. Like other types of replacement therapy, such as giving insulin for the day-to-day control of diabetes, the purpose in either sex is simply to restore hormone levels to near-normality. Estrogen preparations are therefore specifically indicated for post-menopausal and younger women deficient in natural estrogens, as androgens are for testosterone-deficient men. Both are contraindicated in members of the opposite sex, and neither has any place in the preventive therapy of people with normal sex hormone levels. That would initially give rise to excessive concentrations, likely to do more harm than good, and then inhibit the body's natural secretion of sex hormones.

There are strong additional reasons for giving HRT to compensate for estrogen deficiency, especially in younger women. They are at risk – and not only from bone loss – for far longer than the majority who undergo a normal menopause in their fifties. The restoration of estrogen levels protects the cardio-vascular system as well as the bones, reverses atrophic changes in the vulva and vagina (thus relieving dyspareunia), increases libido and gives many women an enhanced sense of wellbeing. These and other potential benefits of HRT do have to be set against possible side-effects, however, notably a gradual rise in the risk of developing breast cancer after 10 years or more of HRT, and the need for regular menstrual bleeding for as long as it continues to be taken, even in old age. Some women, therefore, prefer one of the alternative measures outlined below, which may also be more appropriate for those who did not start taking HRT soon after the menopause and need preventive therapy later in life.

2. *Drugs other than sex hormones* are capable of limiting or reversing bone loss by a variety of mechanisms in women or men, whether deficient in sex hormones or not. Bisphosphonate compounds, calcitonin, and anabolic steroids all act mainly by reducing bone resorption, each in its own distinctive way, as outlined below. The anabolic steroids, which resemble testosterone, also stimulate bone formation, but only fluoride salts can generate substantial quantities of new bone. The use of both is, however, restricted by the danger of long-term side-effects, and fluorides are of questionable value because the extra bone laid down is abnormal in its structure and impaired in strength. This leaves calcitonin and the bisphosphonates as the most acceptable forms of preventive ther-

apy for the many elderly and some younger patients (e.g. those taking long-term corticosteroids in high doses) with excessive bone loss not caused by sex hormone deficiency. They may also be more appropriate for women who do not respond adequately to, cannot tolerate or reject the idea of HRT. In the elderly of both sexes, calcium and vitamin D (or one of its analogues) must now be elevated from the general prophylactic measures, described below, to preventive therapy capable of materially reducing the high risk of hip and other fractures.

3. *General prophylactic measures* – including calcium, vitamin D, physical exertion, and a good mixed diet containing adequate protein – still tend to be underrated by doctor and patient alike, despite growing evidence of their value. These basic requirements are not only vital to promote skeletal development in the young; they also minimize bone losses in adults and should always accompany HRT and other types of preventive therapy.

Additional precautions may be necessary in certain women, to compensate for the various factors that make them peculiarly susceptible to osteoporosis. Except in pregnancy, amenorrhea is almost invariably associated with estrogen deficiency and bone loss, so greater attention should be paid to correcting its more amenable causes, particularly undue thinness in young women. There should also be wider awareness that cigarette smoking reduces the activity of natural estrogens and is therefore likely to be associated with bone loss in younger women and to diminish the effectiveness of HRT, though probably not of other types of preventive therapy, in older women.

SCOPE – AND LIMITATIONS – OF PREVENTIVE THERAPY

Although these drugs and general measures act in various different ways, which largely determine for whom they should be prescribed, they have many features and limitations in common. With the sole exception of fluorides, what they all do most effectively is to conserve existing bone, chiefly by curbing its current rate of loss. They have comparatively little power to restore bone that has already been lost or (fluorides apart) to build up reserves by generating additional bone. None of them can do much more than keep osteoporosis at bay – or for much longer than they continue to be taken regularly. Only the bisphosphonates, whose protective effect declines slowly for a year or more after their withdrawal, can give any protection from future losses. In short, preventive therapy may be best regarded as a holding operation. It seldom adds more than a

Figure 3
'... trabeculae silently destroyed by progressive bone loss...' Almost perfect trabecular framework in the vertebral body of a young adult (a). Many of the horizontal members are lost later in life, with wider separation (and some compensatory thickening) of the vertical components (b). Advanced breakdown of the trabecular framework in a very old woman (c) leaves the few remaining vertical components unsupported – and extremely fracture-prone

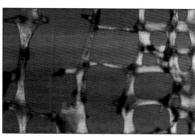
(a)

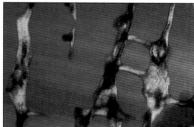
(b)

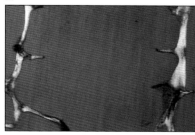
(c)

modest initial bonus to the bone still present when treatment is started – and can do little or nothing to rebuild trabeculae silently destroyed by progressive bone loss (*Figure 3*).

No form of preventive therapy is sufficiently effective, even when given regularly to appropriate patients in recommended dosage, to keep the bone density well above the fracture threshold in every individual at risk, in all parts of their skeletons, or for the rest of their lives. Individual responses to any particular drug and dosage vary quite widely between comparable patients (*Figure 4*) and cannot be relied upon to remain constant during the many years of preventive therapy often required. Hence it is vitally important to monitor the response by regular measurement of the bone density.

Some individuals respond so poorly to an apparently suitable drug – often for no detectable reason – that it has to be changed for another. Others respond well at first but may later relapse into renewed bone loss despite continuing treatment. Sometimes this happens unaccountably, but more often because the patient has not been taking the prescribed dosage, or because additional causes have come into play (such as the menopause, corticosteroid therapy, or old age coupled with inactivity and dietary deficiencies). Certain types of bone loss can also be difficult to control – in patients receiving high doses of corticosteroids, for example, and in some of the rarer, so-called idio-

pathic cases with no known cause for their osteoporosis.

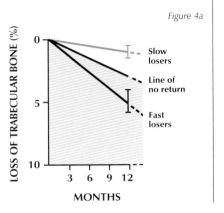
Figure 4a

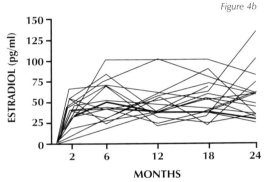
Figure 4b

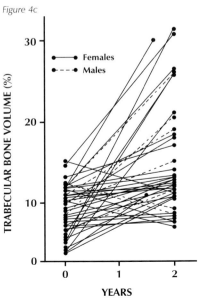
Figure 4c

Figure 4
'Individual responses to any particular drug and dosage vary quite widely ...' Some people lose bone much faster than others (a) and therefore need preventive therapy more urgently – though they may not respond adequately. Serum estradiol levels (b) show marked differences between 20 postmenopausal women receiving the same dose (0.05 mg/24 h) transdermally, as well as marked variability in each individual. Pretreatment differences in trabecular bone volume among 46 osteoporotic patients (c) were greatly and unpredictably exaggerated by 2 years' treatment with sodium fluoride, calcium and vitamin D. Most responded well, and some excellently, while a few deteriorated despite treatment

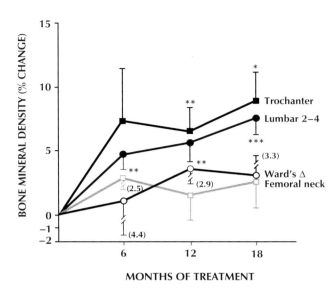

Figure 5
The benefits of preventive therapy also vary '... between one part of the skeleton and another and even between adjacent parts of the same bone'. In response to the bisphosphonate pamidronate, bone density increased significantly in the lumbar vertebrae and the greater trochanter of the femur, among 14 postmenopausal women with osteoporosis, but not in the fracture-prone Ward's triangle or femoral neck. $*p < 0.02$; $**p < 0.005$; $***p < 0.001$. (*See also Figure 16*)

PATTERNS OF PRESCRIBING

These considerations set the framework for all preventive therapy of osteoporosis. Ideally, it ought to be started well before the bone density has fallen to the fracture threshold or the trabecular framework has been irreparably damaged. The choice of preventive therapy can sometimes reflect both the cause and the distribution of the patient's bone loss. Being precipitated by estrogen deficiency, the high turnover and accelerated loss to which the vertebral bodies are particularly prone immediately after the menopause are most appropriately – and effectively – treated with HRT. But preventive therapy cannot always be directed to the cause of osteoporosis, nor need it be. If HRT should be contraindicated for any reason, postmenopausal bone loss may be almost as satisfactorily controlled by a bisphosphonate or calcitonin, for example. More than the prescribing of a particular drug, early diagnosis is the key to preventive therapy, and regular monitoring the measure of its success.

Unless the bone density is monitored at vulnerable sites (typically the forearm, hip and lumbar spine) throughout the period of preventive therapy, persistent or renewed bone loss at any of them would go unnoticed – and the patient continue to be inadequately treated. Should preventive therapy have to be changed or withdrawn, monitoring of the bone density becomes more, not less, important. Otherwise, any recurrence of bone loss would go

The extent to which any type of preventive therapy can bring bone loss under control varies not only from patient to patient, and over time in each individual, but between one part of the skeleton and another (*Figure 5*) and even between adjacent parts of the same bone. These variations probably reflect local differences in rates of bone resorption, outlined in Chapter 3, as much as differences in their response to treatment. Finally, the discontinuation of preventive therapy will be followed by renewed bone loss, which is also variable in severity and distribution, being particularly rapid after withdrawal of HRT. The bone density must therefore continue to be monitored indefinitely. Much of the benefit of several years' preventive therapy may otherwise be lost within a year or two if the underlying causes of bone loss are still silently at work – as they nearly always will be.

unrecognized and consequently unchecked. The long-term efficacy of all preventive therapy depends upon it being promptly adapted to changing needs and continued for as long as the patient remains at risk.

That will usually be lifelong. Patients who have once needed preventive therapy seldom build up sufficient reserves to withstand the renewed bone loss likely to follow its withdrawal. There are only two, rather uncommon situations in which preventive therapy may be discontinued without this penalty: restoration of regular menstrual cycles in a woman of childbearing age, and withdrawal of long-term corticosteroid therapy when it is no longer needed. Even then, other possible causes of bone loss should be considered in such patients and the bone density monitored from time to time if it remains below average. More detailed consideration of the ways in which the various types of preventive therapy act may help to clarify what can reasonably – and what should not – be expected from each of them.

MECHANISMS OF ACTION

All the drugs used to control bone loss act mainly by correcting the underlying imbalance in remodelling (*Figure 6*). Apart from fluorides, they do this chiefly by inhibiting excessive osteoclastic resorption of bone. The outflow of calcium from resorbed bone into the bloodstream is therefore reduced, preventing the excretion of excessive quantities in the urine. The body's calcium balance is further improved by estrogens, testosterone and anabolic steroids, which promote calcium absorption from the digestive tract. Although the last two also stimulate bone formation, and fluorides do so exclusively, the overall picture is biased heavily in favor of antiresorptive drugs acting in various different ways. Between them, they account for well over 90% of all preventive therapy prescribed for osteoporosis at present – though not as a matter of principle. More effective and better tolerated means of stimulating bone formation are badly needed and will no doubt be found in the future. Meanwhile, today's antiresorptive drugs do owe part of their efficacy to an initial increase in bone formation, for which they are only indirectly responsible.

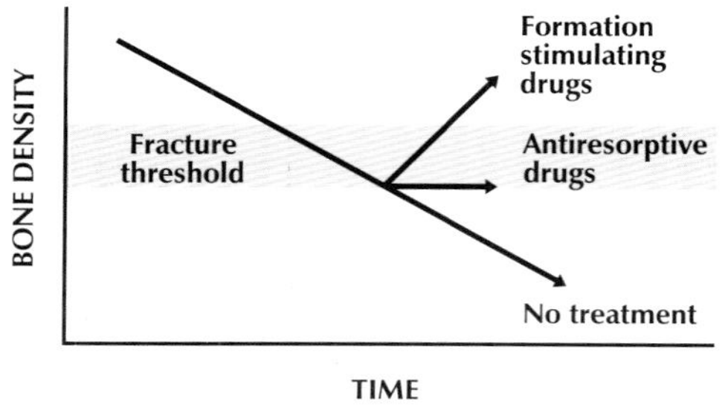

AN INITIAL BONUS

During the first year or more of preventive therapy, HRT and the other drugs that act by reducing resorption typically produce a net gain in bone density instead of simply stemming bone loss. Indeed, the density of trabecular bone typically rises by rather more in the first year than it would have fallen if left untreated (*Figure 7*). At first sight, this initial bonus creates the false impression that estrogens, bisphosphonates and calcitonin must be positively stimulating bone forma-

Figure 6
'All the drugs used to control bone loss act mainly by correcting the underlying imbalance in remodelling.' Most of those currently available are *antiresorptive* and do little more than prevent further deterioration by maintaining the status quo. Only *formation stimulating* drugs could materially increase a low bone density that had already fallen towards or even dropped below the notional fracture threshold, but few are yet available

tion. The real explanation has more to do with the balance of remodelling.

The feedback mechanisms that employ chemical messengers between the osteoclasts and osteoblasts, to match bone formation to the local resorption rate, appear to operate with some delay – in addition to the fact that building new bone takes many times longer than resorbing the old that it eventually replaces. The high turnover and resorption rates that typically follow estrogen withdrawal begin to decline within days of starting HRT, but the enhanced rate at which new bone formation has been vainly attempting to keep pace takes many months to fall gradually into line. There is consequently an appreciable net gain in bone density during the first year of antiresorptive treatment, before the increase tails off during the second (see Figure 7). The rate of bone formation has then declined to match the reduced resorption rate. The only remaining questions are whether such prolonged improvement can be sufficiently explained by temporary imbalance in remodelling, coupled with differences in the timetables of resorption and bone formation – and, if so, whether these factors apply equally to different types of antiresorptive therapy.

However that may be, no appreciable further gains in bone density can be expected after the first 2 years of HRT or most other types of preventive therapy that act by inhibiting resorption. The size of the initial bonus is, in any case, somewhat unpredictable, varying between individuals and not uniform in all areas of trabecular bone. The net gain will usually be greatest where remodelling rates were highest, e.g. in the high-turnover osteoporosis, characteristic of the vertebral bodies following estrogen withdrawal, thanks to the local osteoblasts continuing to form new bone at the brisk tempo previously required. This does not, however, mean that any increase will necessarily be largest where the need is greatest, in terms of low bone density, whether in individuals or particular bones. Nor can there be any certainty that an initial increase will be maintained. Any additional bone is, of course, just as impermanent as the rest of the skeleton, into which it simply becomes incorporated. How well the bone density is maintained thereafter will depend on continuing control of future losses, which each type of preventive therapy exercises in its own distinctive way.

Figure 7
Antiresorptive drugs, such as estradiol, do more than stem bone loss initially. Bone formation typically outstrips the suppressed rate of resorption for the first year or more of treatment, often pushing up the bone density (here in the spine) by at least as much as it would have fallen without treatment. This bonus typically tails off during the second year, as the body's feedback controls reduce bone formation to match the lowered resorption rate

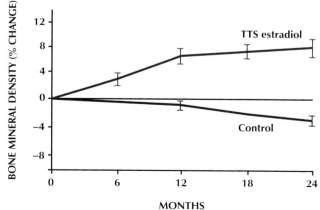

ESTROGENS

Of the three natural estrogens (estrone, estradiol and estriol), estradiol is much the most active in inhibiting resorption, and thus maintaining bone density, followed by estrone. Like the substantial quantities of testosterone also normally present in women, these steroid hormones have functions which differ more than the similarity of their structures might suggest (*Figure 8*). Since estradiol is secreted by the ovarian follicles, as befits its function as the main reproductive estrogen, its production depends on follicular activity during each monthly cycle. It is, therefore, confined to women who are ovulating regularly. Estradiol levels consequently fall more than those of the other estrogens when the menstrual cycle ceases at the menopause or for any other reason (*Figure 9*).

On both these grounds, estradiol is the most logical choice of HRT for the prevention of osteoporosis following the menopause and in younger women with persistent amenorrhea caused by removal or malfunctioning of the ovaries. Estrone would be much less effective at protecting the bones, and estriol relatively inactive. One of the leading HRT preparations (Premarin®, extracted from pregnant mares' urine) nevertheless contains a conjugated mixture of equine estrogens,

Figure 8
Chemical structures of the main steroid sex hormones, all derived from the much-maligned but indispensable cholesterol molecule. Only minimal differences distinguish the three female sex hormones – estrone, estradiol, and estriol, with 1, 2 and 3 hydroxy radicles, respectively – from one another and from the male sex hormone, testosterone. Progesterone also shares the same basic steroidal structure, in which chemically minor modifications make fundamental changes in reproductive and other biological functions

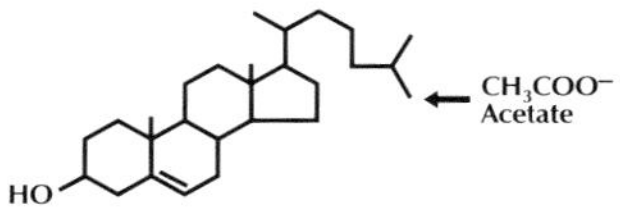

CHOLESTEROL

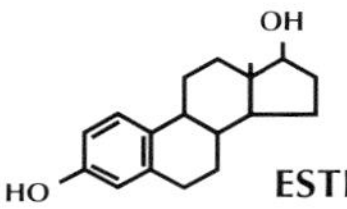

ESTRADIOL

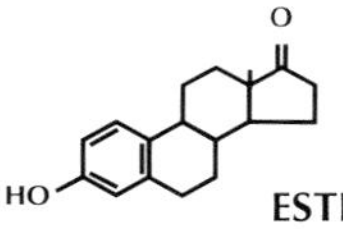

ESTRONE

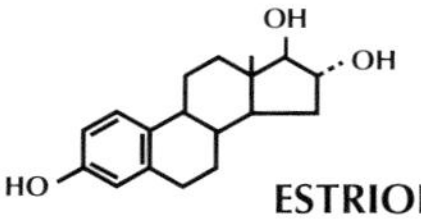

ESTRIOL

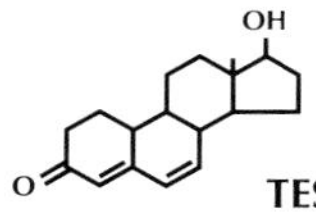

TESTOSTERONE

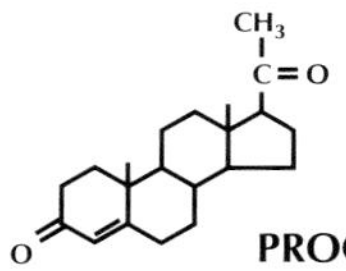

PROGESTERONE

Table 3 The main types of estrogen-containing hormone replacement therapy (HRT).
For HRT preparations containing progestogen, see Table 6

Hormone content	Typical proprietary names *	Dose
Oral preparations		
Conjugated equine estrogens	Premarin	0.625, 1.25 mg
Estradiol valerate	Climaval, Estrace	1, 2 mg
Estradiol valerate	Progynova, Estrace	1, 2 mg
Estradiol	Zumenon, Estrace	2 mg
Piperazine estrone sulfate	Harmogen, Ogen	1.5 mg
Estriol	Ovestin, Estrovis	1 mg
Mixed estrogens	Hormonin	estrone 1.4 mg, estradiol 0.6 mg, and estriol 0.27 mg
Transdermal preparations		
Estradiol	Estraderm (patch), Estraderm	0.025, 0.05, 0.1 mg/24 h
Estradiol	Evorel (patch), Systen	0.05 mg/24 h
Estradiol	Oestrogel (gel)	2.5 mg
Implants		
Estradiol	Estradiol implant, Estrapel	25, 50, 100 mg
Vaginal creams		
Conjugated equine estrogens	Premarin	0.625 mg/g
Estriol	Orthogynest	0.01%
Estriol	Ovestin, Estragard	0.1%
Dienestrol	Ortho-Dienoestrol	0.01%
Vaginal pessaries		
Estradiol	Vagifem, Estrace vaginal	0.025 mg
Estriol	Ortho-Gynest	0.5 mg

* The proprietary names vary from country to country

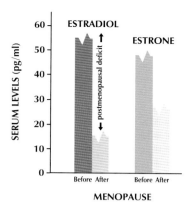

Figure 9
Because estradiol is formed predominantly by ovarian follicles, its serum levels fall more, when ovulation ceases at the menopause, than those of the other estrogens (and testosterone) which continue to be produced. Estradiol is both the most needed and the most effective form of replacement therapy, not only for controlling hot flushes and other menopausal symptoms but also for the long-term prevention of bone loss and cardiovascular disease (*see Figure 10*)

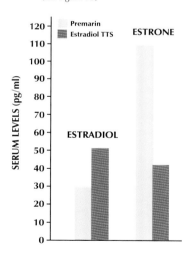

Figure 10
Hormone levels produced by two of the main forms of HRT. The serum levels of estradiol and estrone during long-term treatment with oral conjugated equine estrogens (Premarin) are disproportionate compared with the more physiological levels produced by transdermal absorption from an estradiol skin patch (Estraderm). The relative imbalance between estradiol and estrone levels in patients taking conjugated equine estrogens has three main sources: the nature of the preparation itself, its oral administration, and subsequent metabolic changes (*see Figure 13*)

taken in tablet form. In contrast to its main rival, transdermal absorption of estradiol alone from a skin patch (Estraderm®), conjugated equine estrogens taken by mouth give rise to unbalanced blood levels, exaggerated by the body's own metabolism (*Figure 10*). The pattern of steady transdermal absorption of controlled amounts of estradiol right round the clock comes much closer to the pattern of natural secretion. It also has the advantage of avoiding the vagaries of gastrointestinal absorption, and the unphysiological peak blood levels, with subsequent troughs, that follow each dose of any drug taken by mouth (*Figure 11*).

Clinical trials have, however, shown these oral and transdermal dosage forms to be about equally effective, both in relieving menopausal symptoms and in preventing bone loss. The choice between them (and the other HRT preparations listed in *Table 3*) may, therefore, rest more on differences in their metabolism and side-effects, and perhaps above all on the patient's personal preference.

Many women would rather apply a skin patch (*Figure 12*) twice a week than take a daily tablet, which is harder to remember and more likely to cause gastrointestinal side-effects. Others may prefer tablet taking, perhaps because they have a local skin reaction to the patch or fear that it may sometimes come off without them noticing – and thus interrupt treatment that should be continuous. Some favor an estrogen-containing ointment for application to the vulva and vagina, to relieve irritation, dyspareunia and other local symptoms, while others simply rub it into any convenient area of skin. In either case, estrogens will be absorbed into the bloodstream to produce systemic as well as any local effects. The main disadvantage of this rough-and-ready form of application is that, unlike the controlled delivery from a skin patch at a predetermined rate, the dosage cannot be accurately controlled.

The control of dosage has also proved to be a problem with estrogen implants, which some women prefer because they only need to be inserted at long intervals. Apart from occasional local reactions, the slow release from them is relatively unpredictable and may decline within a few months. Otherwise, the convenience of being able to forget about estrogen administration for many months at a time would have led to much wider use of implants – and may yet do so as their design is further improved.

Although conjugated equine estrogens had the advantage of

being introduced before most other forms of HRT, so that their efficacy and safety have been well established, transdermal estradiol produces similar benefits with significantly less metabolic disturbance. Like all other drugs taken by mouth, conjugated estrogens first have to be absorbed from the stomach, which entails some modification, and then pass immediately to the liver (*Figure 13a*). This hepatic 'first pass' has three important effects:

1) The liver enzymes further modify the conjugated estrogens, contributing to the distorted blood profiles illustrated in *Figure 10*.

2) Exposure to high estrogen concentrations affects the liver's own metabolism, with the favorable and more questionable effects noted in *Table 4*.

3) While most of the estrogen taken orally passes out of the liver, modified or unmodified, into the systemic circulation, much finds its way into the bile and thus re-enters the intestinal tract – only to be reabsorbed and pass through the liver again ... and again (*see Figure 13a*). This recycling contributes to the relatively high local concentrations responsible for some of the gastric and hepatic side-effects of estrogens taken orally.

By contrast, estradiol or any other drug steadily absorbed via the skin (or from an implant) enters the systemic circulation directly, without

passing the liver first, and consequently without producing these potentially adverse effects or the peak concentrations that contribute to them (*Figure 13b*).

Antiresorptive mechanisms of action

Estradiol appears to inhibit bone resorption mainly by counteracting the stimulant action of parathyroid hormone (PTH). In regularly menstruating women, the effects of

Figure 11
Nearly all drugs taken by mouth produce swings in blood concentration, above and below the optimal range (a). The unnecessarily high peaks following each dose may provoke undesirable side-effects, while the subsequent troughs often fall below effective therapeutic levels. Steady transdermal absorption from an Estraderm skin patch (see *Figure 12*) gives estradiol concentrations closer to the optimal level (b) found at mid-cycle in women of child-bearing age

Figure 11a

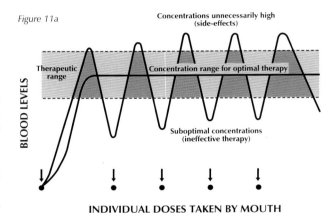

INDIVIDUAL DOSES TAKEN BY MOUTH

Figure 11b

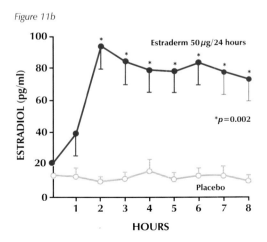

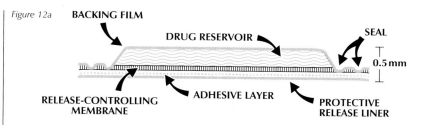

Figure 12a

BACKING FILM
DRUG RESERVOIR
SEAL
0.5 mm
RELEASE-CONTROLLING MEMBRANE
ADHESIVE LAYER
PROTECTIVE RELEASE LINER

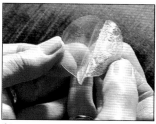

(b)

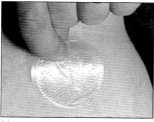

(c)

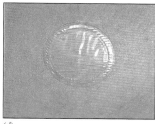

(d)

Figure 12
Transdermal estradiol in principle and practice. The Estraderm skin patch is transparent, flexible and only 0.5 mm thick (a). It comes in three sizes (*see Table 3*), releasing different doses of estradiol from the reservoir, via the controlling membrane and adhesive layer, into the skin, where it is absorbed into the bloodstream. Application simply requires removal of the protective liner (*b*) before sticking the patch (*c*) to hairless skin, usually over the hips or lower abdomen (*d*). Absorption continues for at least 4 days but patches are normally replaced twice weekly

Figure 13
Like all other drugs taken by mouth, conjugated equine estrogens first pass from the stomach to the liver. Estrogens then recirculate between them (*a*), affecting hepatic metabolism, distorting the estrogen profile (*see Figure 10*), and increasing the risk of local hepatic and gastric side-effects. These are largely avoided by transdermal administration of estradiol, which may cause a local skin reaction in some patients but then bypasses the stomach and liver (*b*), without producing high local concentrations

these and other influences on bone remodelling are approximately in balance. When menstruation ceases, at whatever age, estradiol levels fall, leaving PTH relatively free to stimulate resorption. New bone formation cannot then keep pace, unless HRT (or some other antiresorptive drug) is given to counteract the unbridled effect of PTH and thus bring remodelling back into balance. In practice, comparable doses of transdermal estradiol and oral conjugated estrogens are about equally effective in controlling the bone loss resulting from estrogen deficiency in women of any age (*Figure 14*).

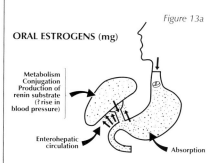

Figure 13a

ORAL ESTROGENS (mg)

Metabolism
Conjugation
Production of renin substrate
(? rise in blood pressure)

Enterohepatic circulation

Absorption

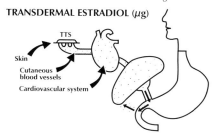

Figure 13b

TRANSDERMAL ESTRADIOL (µg)

TTS
Skin
Cutaneous blood vessels
Cardiovascular system

Neither estradiol nor the other natural estrogens seem able to stimulate the osteoblasts to lay down more new bone – although these cells have been found to possess estradiol receptors. Their function, when activated by the presence of estradiol, may be to stimulate release of a local mediator that exerts feedback control over the osteoclasts, inhibiting their resorptive activity. It is not yet clear whether estrogens or other types of preventive therapy have any influence over the lining cells and osteocytes, scattered throughout the bone substance (*see Figure 3* in Chapter 2), which seem to act like district surveyors, constantly assessing the local situation, and apparently issuing instructions for the local remodelling of bone, in which they play no active part.

Specific estradiol receptors have been identified in numerous organs and tissues, including some that show no obvious signs of deterioration when deprived of the hormone. Receptors in the skin, blood vessels and intestinal wall presumably mediate much or all of the beneficial effect of estrogen replacement, respectively, on skin texture and appearance, in preventing cardiovascular disease, and in promoting the absorption of dietary calcium.

The enhanced mood and wellbeing of many postmenopausal and younger women taking HRT almost certainly reflect its action on estradiol receptors in brain cells, which could well play a part in increasing libido. The estrogen content of HRT, given orally or transdermally, also reverses menopausal changes in the vulva, vagina, breasts and uterus of estrogen-deficient women, heightening sensitivity and sexual responsiveness, relieving dyspareunia, and stimulating the endometrium. These and other tissues retain estradiol receptors long after the menopause, enabling them to respond to local or systemic estrogen replacement even in old age.

TESTOSTERONE

For their transient and relatively simple role in procreation, men are equipped with a predominant sex hormone, testosterone (*see Figure 8*), both to serve reproductive purposes and to endow the male with the physical strength and aggressiveness required to protect and provide for his family.

Since most testosterone is secreted by the testes, their malfunctioning or removal greatly reduces its blood levels. Men with no testicular production are left with low concentrations secreted by the adrenals or derived from the comparatively small amounts of estrogens normally present in the male. Replacement therapy can be given daily by mouth, or in the form of skin patches or long-acting implants. As with estradiol, transdermal absorption is preferable. Skin patches provide steady delivery of measured amounts which avoids both the hepatic first pass and the peak blood levels that follow each oral dose, either of which may provoke side-effects. Absorption from implants also enjoys these advantages, but it cannot yet be equally well controlled or as reliably sustained over many months.

Table 4 Biochemical effects of HRT on liver metabolism	
Lipids	
Total cholesterol	reduced
LDL cholesterol	reduced
HDL cholesterol (protective)	raised
HDL/LDL ratio (high is good)	raised
Clotting factors	
Antithrombin III	reduced
Hypertensive factor	
Renin substrate	raised, especially on oral estrogens

The changes in lipids and clotting factors are considered improvements, HRT tending to reverse the increased risks of cardiovascular and thromboembolic disease in postmenopausal women by restoring cholesterol and antithrombin levels towards premenopausal values.

Increased production of renin substrate could raise the blood pressure, however, particularly in women taking oral (rather than transdermal) HRT.

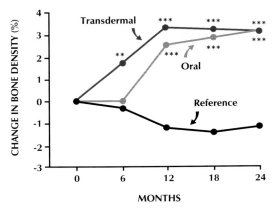

Figure 14
Both transdermal estradiol and oral estrogens increase bone density significantly in postmenopausal women, compared with unabated bone loss in control subjects. Note how the bone density (here in the lumbar spine) rises during the first year or more of treatment, before levelling off in the second.
$**p < 0.01$; $***p < 0.001$ compared with untreated reference cases

Figure 15
Pyrophosphate, naturally present in bone mineral, compared with the three bisphosphonate compounds most commonly used as preventive therapy. The structural similarities lead to the bisphosphonates being 'mistaken' for pyrophosphate and incorporated into bone, which they protect by inhibiting its resorption. These bisphosphonate compounds, and others still being developed, each have distinctive properties determined by the rest of their molecular structure

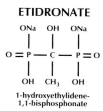

INORGANIC PYROPHOSPHATE

CLODRONATE

Dichloromethylene-1,1-bisphosphonate

ETIDRONATE

1-hydroxyethylidene-1,1-bisphosphonate

PAMIDRONATE

3-amino-1-hydroxypropylidene-1,1-bisphosphonate

Compared with estradiol, testosterone has been the subject of rather less detailed study of its normal functions, the ill-effects of its deficiency or the value of replacement therapy. Specific testosterone receptors – and therefore, by implication, actions – have, however, been identified on the cells of many different tissues and organs. The fact that testosterone deficiency produces few outward signs should not be taken to imply that those actions are unimportant, though some may be comparatively trivial. Its main effect on bone, resembling that of estradiol in women, is to curb resorption by opposing the action of PTH. Its stimulation of bone formation is less pronounced, probably acting directly on the osteoblasts. Testosterone also aids calcium absorption, and often increases virility. It is, therefore, the logical form of preventive therapy for osteoporosis in men of any age who have abnormally low blood levels. It cannot restore their fertility, though, any more than estrogen replacement does in women, and recent claims of cardiovascular benefit have yet to be substantiated.

BISPHOSPHONATES

The bisphosphonates are a family of synthetic compounds, mostly developed for the detergent industry, some of which have been modified to inhibit bone resorption. They all have a characteristic chemical grouping in common, consisting of twin phosphorus atoms symmetrically linked to a single carbon atom (P–C–P), resembling the pyrophosphate linkage via an oxygen molecule (P–O–P) which forms part of the normal bone mineral, hydroxyapatite. By virtue of this structural similarity, bisphosphonates given as preventive therapy for osteoporosis become firmly attached to the internal surfaces of trabecular bone all over the body. The differences between the various compounds now available (*Figure 15*) are determined by the other parts of their molecules. When one of them has become incorporated into the surface of the bone mineral, it acts as a protective coating. This appears to prevent the osteoclasts from recognizing the internal bone surfaces as targets for resorption. Indeed, the newer bisphosphonate, alendronate, seems to act preferentially at active resorption sites – just where it is most desirable to prevent bone loss.

By blocking the first stage of remodelling, wherever it would normally be taking place, bisphosphonates prevent the entire process. They also appear to reduce the number of osteoclasts engaged in bone resorption and perhaps inhibit their activity, though such effects could be secondary to the reduced demand for these functions. Like other workers made redundant during a period of recession, osteoclasts may simply disperse when there is no work for them to do, leaving a skeleton crew to attend to any emergency repairs that may be required.

That some osteoclasts remain on call in bisphosphonate-treated bone is clear from the fact that fractures heal quite normally, probably because the fractured bone surfaces are unprotected. Whatever the precise mechanisms involved, the ability of bisphosphonates to protect undamaged trabecular bone from resorption – and thus from fractures – has been amply demonstrated in controlled trials (*Figure 16*) and endorsed by growing experience in clinical practice. Bisphosphonate therapy does require close monitoring and quite rigorous precautions, however, and some uncertainties remain about its suitability for long-term preventive therapy.

The main precautions required concern dosage. Because the characteristic P–C–P linkage binds bisphosphonates to bone mineral for long periods, any overdosage can have a cumulative effect. Bisphosphonates then demineralize – and consequently weaken – the osteoporotic bone they are intended to protect, producing an osteomalacia-like condition. To avoid this, all bisphosphonate compounds should be given in low doses and/or intermittently, often for spells of a few weeks or months separated by treatment-free intervals of similar duration. Monitoring of the bone density is vital, to ensure that an optimal balance is maintained between the desired control of resorption and the risk of demineralization.

Two further provisos must be noted. First, since bisphosphonates protect trabecular bone, in particular, by preventing its regular remod-

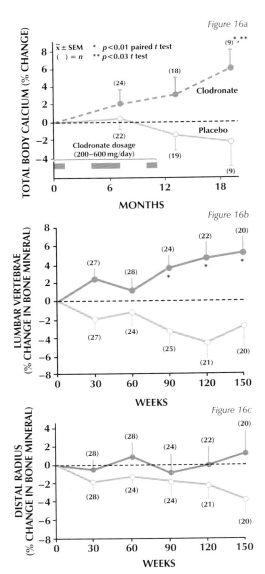

Figure 16a

Figure 16b

Figure 16c

Figure 16
Bisphosphonates as preventive therapy. Intermittent clodronate treatment over 12 months increased the total body calcium of osteoporotic patients and continued to inhibit bone resorption for at least 6 months after its withdrawal – in contrast to the persistent bone loss among placebo-treated patients (a). The benefit is not uniform throughout the skeleton, however, typically being greater in the trabecular bone of the lumbar spine (b) than in the distal radius (c), as shown by a study of intermittent etidronate therapy. (See also Figure 5)

elling, their prolonged use eventually leads to protected bone outliving its normal lifespan. This raises fundamental questions that have yet to be definitively answered:

1) How necessary is it to the health and strength of normal bone for it to be regularly remodelled?

2) What, if anything, would eventually go wrong with bone if nature's normal schedule of renovations were too long deferred?

3) And, if so, how long would be too long?

By inhibiting resorption, bisphosphonates prevent all subsequent stages of remodelling – which is the sole mechanism that enables bone to adapt, for better or worse, to changing circumstances. Bone that was prevented from regularly regenerating itself over many years would eventually be bound to lose much of its capacity to respond positively to exertion, or any other stimulus, by strengthening its own structure. Without firm evidence, it can only be surmised that the osteocytes in unregenerated bone may gradually degenerate and decline in numbers, as they do in old age. Once the mineralized protein matrix had passed its 'renew by' date, the strength and resilience of trabecular bone could well decline, until it became 'fatigued' and fracture-prone, like aging metal. Such changes may already contribute to the friability of bone in extreme old age. The preservation of younger bone in a way that prevented its regular regeneration could have similar effects.

How important these reservations about the long-term effects of bisphosphonate therapy may prove to be in practice remains uncertain. Neither the mechanisms of bone remodelling nor the reasons for it are fully understood. There is no known biological example of a living species with 'fossilized' bone that does not undergo regular renovation, and clinical experience is based on little more than a decade of prescribing bisphosphonates. Favorable though most of that experience has been, it can give only provisional reassurance about their longer-term suitability and safety in the many patients whose bone loss needs to be controlled for several decades.

CALCITONINS

The calcitonins are natural hormones, present in animals and fish, with slight species' differences in their chemical structure. In mammals they are secreted into the bloodstream by the thyroid gland and play an ill-defined part in the complex control of bone remodelling by inhibiting resorption.

Human calcitonin does not appear to be deficient in osteoporotic patients, so its use cannot be regarded as hormone replacement. Nor does the thyroid appear to produce extra calcitonin to curb bone loss. Its inhibitory effect on bone resorption can, however, be exploited by giving additional amounts. This hormone *supplementation* does not rely solely on human or even mammalian calcitonin (usually obtained from pigs). The remarkably similar compounds produced by fish for other purposes are active in man, and salmon calcitonin has proved to be both effective and well tolerated as preventive therapy for osteoporosis.

Calcitonins would probably be employed more widely were it not for the high cost of their purification or synthesis and the fact that none of them are active by mouth. As polypeptide (i.e. protein-type) hormones, all calcitonins are rapidly broken down into their constituent peptides and amino acids by the digestive system, and thus inactivated. They therefore need to be given either by injection or by spray inhalation into the nose for direct absorption (via its lining membrane) into the bloodstream.

Of the preparations studied in detail, synthetic human and salmon calcitonins have been shown to prevent osteoporotic bone loss by inhibiting osteoclast activity, and thus to increase and then stabilize the bone density, and so reduce the risk of fracture (*Figure 17*). Doubts have, however, been expressed about the long-term efficacy of calcitonin therapy, on two main grounds. Even minor deviations from the protein structure of the human hormone could provoke an immune response, with antibody production blocking its action. Second, the giving of extra calcitonin might desensitize its specific receptors in bone, making still higher concentrations necessary to obtain the desired effect. Fortunately, neither of these theoretical objections seems to create insuperable problems in practice. The beneficial effects of calcitonin therapy, which include unusually rapid relief of the bone pain associated with osteoporotic fractures (particularly in the vertebral bodies), therefore have to be

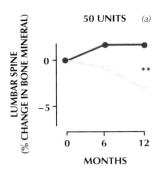
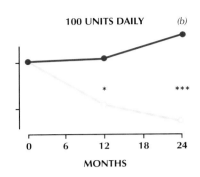

weighed mainly against its high cost and the absence of an oral dosage form. It remains to be seen how well these practical disadvantages of an effective form of preventive therapy can be overcome.

ANABOLIC STEROIDS

The anabolic steroids are synthetic analogues of testosterone, created by modifying its structure. They were first developed for medical use, to forestall muscle loss or aid its restoration in patients with wasting diseases. The intention was to eliminate the virilizing effects of testosterone while retaining its desired 'anabolic' functions. The word (derived from the Greek for 'ascent') implies the building up of larger organic molecules, particularly the structural protein of muscle and bone matrix, from smaller components – in this case amino acids. The original aim of stimulating that process has been successfully attained in today's anabolic steroids (*Figure 18*). It has not so far proved possible to rid these modified hormones of all virilizing actions, however,

Figure 17
Calcitonin as preventive therapy. Nasal inhalation of salmon calcitonin (50 units, 5 days per week) by recently postmenopausal women produced a modest initial increase in the mineral density of the lumbar spine, followed by stabilization, compared with continuing losses among untreated women (a). Larger doses (100 units) taken daily sustained the beneficial effect over 2 years (b). *$p < 0.01$; **$p < 0.001$; ***$p < 0.0001$ compared with untreated controls

Figure 18
Anabolic steroids as treatment for osteoporosis. Sustained increase in total body calcium produced by stanozolol over a 2-year period, compared with placebo (a). The striking effect of nandrolone, alone or combined with calcium and calcitriol, on the vertebral mineral density of postmenopausal women, compared with continuing loss in control subjects before stabilizing at a lower level on calcium and calcitriol (b)

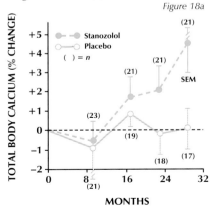

and their medical value is restricted by these and other side-effects.

The use of anabolic steroids cannot be regarded as hormone replacement, except conceivably in testosterone-deficient men, for whom testosterone itself would be preferable. They are, therefore, used more for treating established osteoporosis in older patients than for long-term prevention of bone loss earlier in life. Although their virilizing effects – facial hair growth, lowering of the voice, and male-type body configuration – mean that they are contraindicated in menopausal and younger women, they may be given to either sex later in life. Even then, caution is necessary because, in addition to virilization, anabolic steroids affect liver function, distorting blood lipid levels. Excessive or unduly prolonged dosage may seriously damage the liver, increase the risk of atherosclerosis in the arteries, and may stimulate overdevelopment of the heart muscle.

Medical caution coupled with the banning of anabolic steroids by sports' authorities has done little to restrain their widespread misuse (which extends to black market supplies of questionable composition and purity) by weightlifters, body-builders, and athletes. Intent on muscle building in the hope of improving their competitive performance, they commonly neglect the dangers of taking excessive doses, often unsupervised, over long periods. By drawing attention to the hazards of anabolic steroids, including some early deaths from liver disease, these practices have highlighted the need for proper control of their prescribing, in carefully controlled dosage and, where possible, for limited periods.

On the other hand, the prompt action of anabolic steroids in stimulating formation of new bone as well as inhibiting resorption and promoting calcium absorption gives them a valuable place in the preventive therapy of more severe osteoporosis, especially in older patients with a low bone density and/or a high rate of loss, which needs to be brought rapidly under control. The overall effect can be quite striking, improving the appearance, increasing drive and creating a sense of wellbeing in addition to strengthening the bones and muscles. Frail patients often become more active as well as physically more robust, are therefore less likely to fall, and have more muscle and soft tissues to control and cushion the impact if they do.

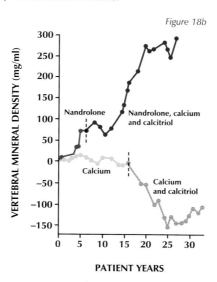

Figure 18b

The balance between these beneficial actions and the undesired effects of anabolic steroids depends on their chemical structure and route of administration as well as dosage. The 17α-alkylated steroids (e.g. stanozolol) are active by mouth but tend to have undesirable hepatic and lipid effects, partly resulting from their first pass through the liver (see Figure 13a). These changes can, however, be minimized by giving a 17β-esterified steroid (such as nandrolone decanoate) by injection so that it avoids the first-pass effect. This only needs to be administered at intervals of 3–4 weeks, which should improve compliance and certainly facilitates low-dose maintenance therapy. Anabolic steroids differ from HRT and most other forms of preventive therapy in that their withdrawal is less likely to provoke an immediate resurgence of bone loss. Small and/or widely spaced doses should, therefore, maintain the benefits of an initial course of more intensive treatment, and keep the risk of virilizing and other side-effects to a minimum.

FLUORIDE SALTS

Fluorides deserve consideration as the sole form of preventive therapy that acts primarily by stimulating formation of new bone. Although capable of producing a considerable, sustained increase in the mineral density of trabecular bone (Figure 19), they have yet to find a major place in the prevention or treatment of osteoporosis. Because fluoride salts need to be given in doses larger than those required to strengthen and protect the teeth, they are more likely to cause gastrointestinal disturbance and other side-effects. Excessive or unduly prolonged dosage produces permanent mottling of the teeth in children (who are fortunately not likely to need it to protect their bones). It may aggravate joint symptoms in arthritic patients, and can cause painful inflammation of the plantar fascia (in the sole of the foot). Prolonged or heavy overdosage at any age results in the pathological condition known as fluorosis. This consists of bone overgrowth with skeletal abnormalities and is seen in parts of India and other countries, where the natural fluoride content of the local water is exceptionally high.

To prevent such ill effects, yet ensure that enough fluoride is given to increase the bone density, its therapeutic use calls for strict control

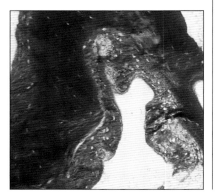

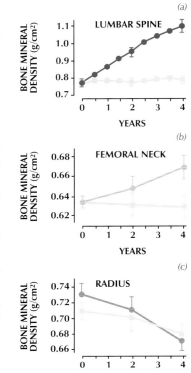

Figure 19
Fluoride as treatment for osteoporosis. Progressive increase in the bone mineral content of trabecular bone in the lumbar spine (a) and femoral neck (b) over 4 years among osteoporotic patients given 75 mg sodium fluoride daily (●), compared with those receiving placebo and calcium (■). The fluoride-induced increase in trabecular bone is unlikely to be matched by increased strength. In patients given the same treatment, the mainly cortical bone in the shaft of the radius failed to benefit (c)

Figure 20
So-called woven bone, typically of normal mineral content but substandard strength, generated by fluoride therapy. Its characteristic 'woven' appearance, with irregularly scattered osteocytes and somewhat lighter blue staining, overlies lamellar bone (stained deeper blue) of normal appearance and strength. The red-stained surface areas are newly formed osteoid, not yet mineralized with fluoro- rather than hydroxyapatite

of dosage and monitoring of the response. The new bone laid down will nevertheless be abnormal in two important respects: it forms a diffuse mass where there is most room for it, over the internal surfaces of trabecular bone (*Figure 20*), and is mineralized with fluoroapatite instead of the normal hydroxyapatite.

So-called 'woven' bone, induced by fluoride therapy, consequently lacks the chemical composition, the physical strength and the latticework structure that give normal trabecular bone such a favorable weight-to-strength ratio. For these reasons, the increased mineral content may not reduce the fracture risk correspondingly. The best that can be expected of fluoride therapy at present is that enough of the additional bone may be incorporated into the normal trabecular structure, in the course of subsequent remodelling, to increase its strength. Even then, long-term HRT, bisphosphonates or some other antiresorptive therapy may be needed to maintain its increased density.

Figure 21
Calcium and vitamin D (cholecalciferol) as fracture prevention in old age. Over the 3 years of study, the high risk of hip fracture among elderly osteoporotic patients was reduced by nearly 30% in the group given daily supplements of 1200 mg calcium and 800 IU (20 µg) cholecalciferol, compared with those taking placebo. Non-vertebral fractures (including those of the hip) were reduced by nearly 25%. These statistically significant results are representative of several recent trials that have demonstrated the preventive value of calcium and vitamin D in old age

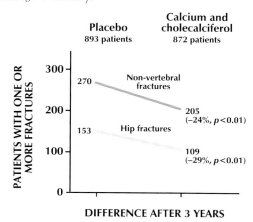

CALCIUM ...

After years of debate about the preventive value, or otherwise, of supplementary calcium (with or without vitamin D), recent studies leave no real doubt that a high enough intake can reduce both the rate of bone loss and the risk of fracture in old people prone to, or already suffering from, osteoporosis (*Figure 21*). This is not merely a matter of compensating for inadequate dietary calcium or the decline in its absorption that normally follows the menopause and accompanies aging. Increasing the intake sufficiently to raise the calcium concentration in the blood produces a feedback effect, which lowers PTH production; the osteoclasts are then less strongly stimulated to resorb calcium from the bones.

To be sure of reducing bone loss significantly in an elderly postmenopausal woman, an old person of either sex or anyone else prone to osteoporosis, the daily calcium intake from all sources probably needs to exceed 1500 mg, equivalent to nearly two-and-a-half pints (or one-and-a-half liters) of milk, every single day. There is no danger of overdosage above this level, but lower intakes seem to be of disproportionately little preventive value. A total of 1000 mg a day (which exceeds the recommended daily intake for a younger adult) cannot be relied upon to produce two-thirds of the protective effect of 1500 mg, and may be insufficient to curb bone loss in the elderly. This seems to be the main reason why many past studies, based on lower (or questionable) daily intakes, failed to demonstrate the efficacy of extra calcium in curbing bone loss, either among postmenopausal women or in the elderly, whose normal diet may well contain less than 500 mg of calcium each day.

Trebling or quadrupling such a low calcium intake to be sure that it exceeds 1500 mg a day calls for major dietary changes and/or supplements. Even that will not be as effective as HRT or other forms of preventive therapy, but calcium has the advantages of being cheap, readily available, well tolerated and free of serious side-effects. It deserves greater recognition not only for its vital part in building strong bones, but both as a first line of defence against osteoporosis and as an adjunct to all forms of preventive therapy. There are no circumstances in which remodelling can be expected to maintain the mineral content of bone without adequate supplies of this vital building material.

Much or all of a higher calcium intake can usefully come from a diet rich in milk and/or yoghurt, from which calcium is particularly well absorbed. Green vegetables, other calcium-rich foods, and even hard water can help in attaining the daily total. Soya preparations rival dairy products in their calcium content and aid its absorption by virtue of the so-called plant estrogens they contain. These compounds have been shown to distort the menstrual cycle of regular soya-bean eaters by

as much as 2 days in each 28-day cycle – which may well mean that they could also have some HRT-like effect in alleviating menopausal hot flushes. They may even reduce post-menopausal bone resorption to some extent. But soya beans are no more a panacea for osteoporosis than dairy products. The crucial test for such foodstuffs, as for calcium supplements, is how much they can contribute to the total intake from all sources, and whether HRT or some other form of preventive therapy may be needed to ensure that calcium is not only well absorbed but also deposited in the bones.

. . . AND VITAMIN D

Daily vitamin D supplements are also likely to be required by many people at risk, unless their diet is unusually rich in the milk fats and fish oils which are its most abundant sources, or they are regularly exposed to sufficient sunlight to synthesize enough in their own skin (see Figure 23). But both animal fats and sunbathing are now frowned upon as health hazards. The total intake of vitamin D, which may well be declining in the population as a whole, must often fall below daily requirements. Yet there are sound reasons for ensuring that they should be satisfied throughout life. As noted earlier, vitamin D is indispensable not only for maximal absorption of calcium from food but also for optimal mineralization of bone, thus preventing rickets in children and the under-mineralization of adult bone (osteomalacia) which can accompany osteoporosis in adults, further weakening the bones. Its prevention becomes especially important from middle age onwards, when absorption of vitamin D (as well as calcium) slowly declines.

All postmenopausal women and elderly people, many of whose diets are also deficient, would be well advised to take daily vitamin D supplements, either as capsules or in the form of cod or halibut liver oil. The recommended daily dose should always be strictly adhered to, since excess vitamin D will do no extra good and can be harmful, even to the bones. Studies of the active metabolite 1,25 dihydroxy-vitamin D (the form known as calcitriol, which circulates throughout the body) have revealed some advantages over the natural vitamin. It may therefore be preferred for preventive therapy, especially in old age.

OTHER DIETARY APPROACHES

Among other dietary measures of potential value in the prevention or treatment of osteoporosis, a case can be made for giving extra phosphates as the essential counterpart of calcium in bone mineral. While some trials have shown apparent benefits, a balanced diet is not normally deficient in phosphate, and there is as yet no proof that supplements would be of much value in reducing bone loss or promoting full mineralization.

A wider-ranging proposal has recently been based on the observation that most human diets tend to be tilted slightly to the acid side of neutral. This could have the effect of slowly leaching alkaline salts from the body, and thus play a part in the slow decline from peak bone mass and contribute to accelerated bone loss of all kinds. No more than slight reduction in acidic and acid-forming foods, plus extra milk, would be needed to correct the balance. Over a lifetime, the cumulative effect of quite small changes of this kind should improve the body's overall calcium balance, though they would be nowhere near powerful enough to contend with the major causes of accelerated bone loss – or correct their consequences.

EXERCISE AND SPINAL POSTURE

Exercise strengthens the bones exposed to weight-bearing or other stresses, both by inhibiting resorption and by stimulating some new bone formation. It appears to do this most effectively in people with normal sex hormone levels (or taking HRT or anabolic steroids). Not too much should be expected of exercise alone. Amenorrheic ballet dancers with low estrogen levels can become fracture prone in their late teens or twenties, when their bone mass should be near its peak, despite their exceptionally intensive exercise routines. By contrast, the bone mass of male athletes, weightlifters and long-distance runners, who are most unlikely to be testosterone deficient, is generally above average for their age and sex. In addition to maintaining bone strength, regular exercise should further reduce the fracture risk in old age by keeping the muscles strong and improving coordination, thus reducing the chances of falling.

Postural training and exercises may also help to minimize – or defer – the development of a dowager's hump in postmenopausal women and reduce the risk of compression fractures in the lumbar spine. The most effective measure is undoubtedly HRT to prevent accelerated bone loss from the vertebral bodies following estrogen withdrawal, but that is not the sole determinant of spinal fractures. Any increase in the normal curvature of the thoracic spine, or the subjection of the lumbar region to ill-advised bending and lifting, puts additional loading on the vertebral bodies, aggravating the risk of compression fractures that is inherent in their anatomy (*Figure 22*). Early intervention is therefore required. Yet the vertebral bone loss that predictably follows the menopause seldom receives any preventive attention before it has caused vertebral fractures, manifested in spinal deformity that may be not only disfiguring but also painful and disabling. Belated attempts at treatment may then take the form of braces, supports or 'corrective' exercises of uncertain value with which few patients persevere.

It may be better to think in terms of long-term prevention, starting in childhood. The Victorians were probably on the right track when they sought to improve 'deportment' – in a way that now attracts derision – by making schoolgirls walk round with books balanced on their heads. Many of today's girls, especially those who are already round-shouldered in their teens, could benefit from a more modern form of postural training, coupled with exercises, while their spines are still young and adaptable. Increased understanding of the preventive value of an upright posture and

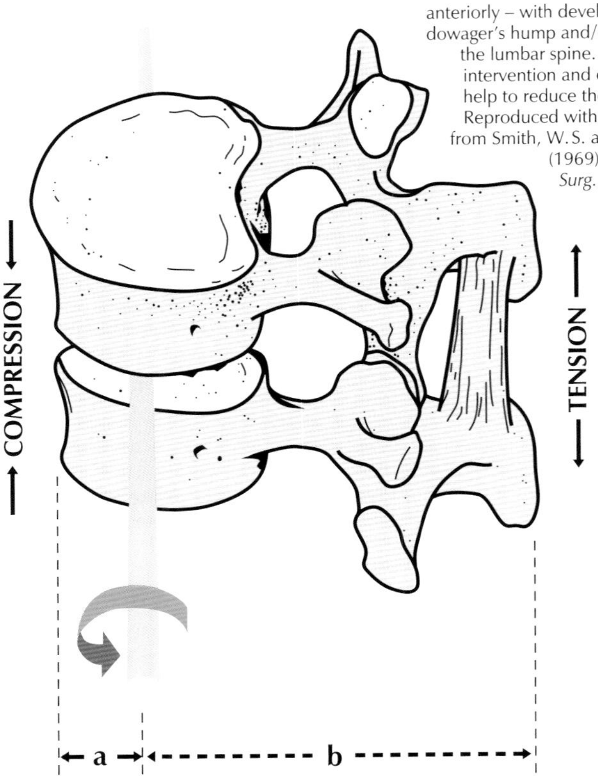

Figure 22
How human anatomy makes the vertebral bodies prone to (anterior) compression fractures. The spine flexes and extends about axes that pass roughly through the centers of the intervertebral discs. Since these axes are about 4 times nearer the front (a) than the back (b) of the vertebrae, spinal flexion compresses the vertebral bodies anteriorly, because there is a little give in the interspinous ligament posteriorly. Hence the tendency for osteoporotic vertebral bodies to become crushed anteriorly – with development of a dowager's hump and/or flattening of the lumbar spine. Early postural intervention and exercises may help to reduce these risks. Reproduced with permission from Smith, W. S. and Kaufer, H. (1969). *J. Bone Joint Surg.*, **51A**, 239–54

strong spinal muscles from youth onwards could help to prevent the upper back from rounding in early middle age and gradually subsiding into a dowager's hump following the menopause. That all-too-familiar picture, often associated with lumbar vertebral fractures, appreciable height loss and distorted posture, ought no longer to be accepted fatalistically, any more than the vertebral bone loss that underlies it is now inevitable. Postural training and regular exercises for the spine might usefully accompany HRT and there may be an even stronger case for them in the many middle-aged women whose bone loss still goes unchecked by preventive therapy of any kind.

PERSONAL PRESCRIBING – THE PATIENT'S PREROGATIVE

The selection of the most suitable form of preventive therapy, and the most appropriate ancillary measures, depends on matching the foregoing methods to the needs of each person at risk. Medical prescribing will clearly be guided mainly by such factors as the patient's age and sex, the probable causes of her or his bone loss, the efficacy and safety of the treatment proposed and, ultimately, by the response. That can only be judged by monitoring the bone density because, however closely preventive therapy is tailored to each individual's material needs, however favorable the trial results in comparable cases, there are many possible reasons – from the purely objective to the highly subjective – why the response in particular individuals or bones may be less than satisfactory.

Objectively, bone loss may not be adequately controlled by an apparently suitable drug taken regularly in what would normally be appropriate dosage, or treatment

may have to be reduced or withdrawn because of potentially serious side-effects. Not all patients respond predictably. Subjectively, some may not be sufficiently convinced of the need for long-term preventive therapy, or of its safety, to overcome their reservations about taking drug treatment daily for years on end. Objections to the unnaturalness of HRT, dislike of a particular preparation, or fear of possible side-effects can result in poor compliance or even complete withdrawal of preventive therapy – of which the doctor may not be aware.

Such prejudices and fears are the patient's prerogative. The doctor can no longer expect to be the sole arbiter of what is best for each individual. Long-term preventive therapy therefore calls for exceptionally close and continuing collaboration, in an atmosphere of mutual trust, based on something like the following guidelines.

THE RECENTLY MENOPAUSAL WOMAN, WHATEVER HER AGE

Since the high turnover and rapid resorption of trabecular bone that follow a natural, premature or surgical menopause are induced by withdrawal of estradiol, HRT is the most logical choice of preventive therapy. Yet replacement therapy is not a panacea for postmenopausal bone loss. To be fully effective, HRT needs to be accompanied by appropriate general measures (*Figure 23*) and continued for many years. Yet most menopausal women start taking HRT for short-term reasons that

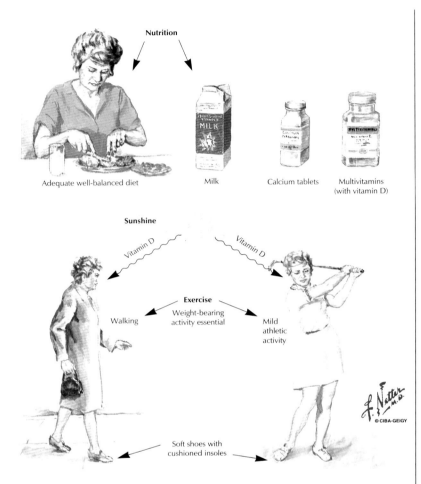

Nutrition

Adequate well-balanced diet   Milk   Calcium tablets   Multivitamins (with vitamin D)

Sunshine

Vitamin D   Vitamin D

Exercise

Walking   Weight-bearing activity essential   Mild athletic activity

Soft shoes with cushioned insoles

Figure 23
HRT is the most logical choice of preventive therapy to compensate for estrogen withdrawal at the menopause – whether surgical or natural, whenever it occurs. But general measures should not be neglected. A well-balanced diet containing sufficient protein, with supplements of calcium and vitamin D (and/or exposure to sunlight), should be accompanied by regular weight-bearing exercise – for which HRT and other forms of preventive therapy cannot adequately substitute

have little or nothing to do with long-term protection from a future risk of osteoporosis. Control of hot flushes or other acute symptoms of estrogen deprivation is by far the commonest motive. This is hardly a reliable way of selecting those in need of HRT to prevent bone loss – or of ensuring that they continue it for long enough to protect them from fractures in old age.

Although the immediate rate of bone loss is loosely related to the severity of menopausal symptoms, individual differences in the responsiveness of the blood vessels play a major part in determining which menopausal women develop hot flushes. At best, the severity of flushes provides only a rough indicator of estrogen deficiency and thus of the short-term need for HRT. Such symptoms are not a reliable guide to the risk of becoming seriously osteoporotic later in life or to the long-term need for preventive therapy.

The lesson is plain. Unless estrogen-deficient women have their bone density determined, the odds are heavily loaded against those most at risk from osteoporosis receiving the long-term preventive therapy they need. They deserve better – in two senses: first, as members of by far the largest group prone to osteoporosis, including the great majority of those who will eventually sustain disabling fractures, and, second, because HRT for women who are estrogen-deficient for any reason is among the most effective forms of preventive therapy yet found for any type of osteoporosis. Each and every one of them should therefore have easy access not only to densitometry but also to the information and advice necessary for her and her doctor to reach rational and mutually acceptable decisions about the most appropriate type of preventive therapy. Some of the key factors to be considered are summarized in Table 5.

In weighing up the pros and cons of HRT, its additional benefits in preventing cardiovascular disease deserve particular attention. In this respect too, HRT ranks among the most effective prophylactic measures yet found, apparently giving postmenopausal and other estrogen-deficient women about as much protection from heart attacks, strokes and other cardiovascular disorders as the combined benefits of not smoking and reducing obesity, cholesterol, high blood pressure and other risk factors.

These advantages of HRT heavily outweigh the gradual rise in breast cancer after 10 years or more of continuous therapy, the evidence for which comes almost exclusively from patients taking oral preparations. Since transdermal estradiol was generally introduced within the last decade, no evidence is yet available about any longer-term effect it may have on the breast cancer rate. However, the risk can be minimized by regular mammography and/or breast examination, as now recommended for all women in this age group. Those taking long-term HRT should already be having regular check-ups, which may be the main reason why more breast cancers are diagnosed among them. The prompt treatment that follows their early diagnosis could also help to explain the relatively small risk of HRT patients dying from the disease. In other words, the fact that these effects are observed in women taking HRT does not necessarily mean that the estrogen treatment itself is wholly responsible for them.

Table 5 Guidelines for decision-making about preventive therapy

Be alert to relevant risk factors, past and present:

Prolonged amenorrhea
Premature or surgical menopause
Corticosteroid therapy
Testosterone deficiency
Postmenopausal status
Old age
Prolonged immobility
Fractures (especially if recurrent and caused by minimal trauma)
Development of dowager's hump and/or back pain

Plus contributory factors: family history, heavy smoking or drinking, lack of exercise, calcium (and/or vitamin D) deficiency

If osteoporosis suspected, measure bone density:

Densitometry, preferably by DXA, of lumbar vertebrae, forearm bones, and hip region

If bone density low (and/or falling rapidly), consider most suitable type of preventive therapy, taking account of age, sex, patient's preference, and any specific indications and contraindications, selecting from:

Hormone replacement (estrogen or testosterone)
Bisphosphonates
Calcitonin
Anabolic steroids
Fluoride salts
Calcium, vitamin D (or calcitriol)

Plus: general measures, and avoidance of adverse factors (see Table 2)

Monitor patient at regular intervals throughout period of preventive therapy and after its eventual withdrawal, particularly checking that:

Treatment taken as prescribed
No unacceptable side-effects
Bone density well maintained

If not, consider adjusting dosage or changing to alternative form of preventive therapy.

That question should be gradually clarified, by more long-term studies of patients taking HRT in transdermal or oral form, combining cyclical progestogen with estrogen replacement.

Ways may yet be found to reduce or even eliminate any added risk of breast cancer in patients taking HRT. Meanwhile, whether a postmenopausal or younger estrogen-deficient woman is prepared to accept that she may be running such a risk if she continues to take HRT for more than 10 years may depend as much on her family history and personal feelings as on the rather sketchy statistics so far available. For some postmenopausal women, anxiety about the possibility of developing breast cancer may outweigh the numerically greater benefits of preventing osteoporosis and cardiovascular disease. Others may take the opposite view, supported by the statistical evidence – though not necessarily for that reason. Logical or illogical as they may be, such decisions must remain the patient's prerogative.

THE NEED FOR PROGESTOGENS – AND MENSTRUATION

For the majority of menopausal women who have not undergone hysterectomy, the major stumbling block to taking HRT is not so much a matter of life and death as the inconvenience of continuing to menstruate. Since this is probably the commonest reason for refusing HRT or discontinuing it prematurely, the need for regular menstrual

bleeds needs to be explained. Giving estrogens by any route stimulates the endometrial cells that line the uterus, mimicking the proliferation produced by natural estradiol secretion during the first 2 weeks of a normal menstrual cycle (known as the proliferative phase for that reason). If estrogen stimulation continues unopposed, it eventually leads to pathologically sustained proliferation – with an enhanced risk of some endometrial cells undergoing cancerous change.

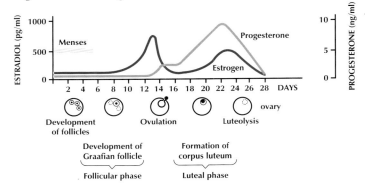

Hysterectomy obviously eliminates that risk. There appears to be no compelling reason why a woman of any age who has had her uterus removed should not take unopposed estrogen replacement therapy indefinitely. Indeed, some middle-aged women undergo hysterectomies so that they can take HRT without continuing to menstruate. In all menopausal women with an intact uterus, however, estrogen replacement needs to be accompanied by a progestogen during the luteal phase of each menstrual cycle (Figure 24), which normally follows ovulation in women of childbearing age and culminates in menstrual bleeding.

Figure 24
'Adding a progestogen to estrogen replacement therapy for 10–14 days each month mimics the natural patterns of progesterone secretion and has much the same effects – precipitating menstrual bleeding and thus virtually eliminating the risk of endometrial cancer.' This can be achieved in practice by taking a progestogen daily by mouth or, more conveniently, by exchanging an estradiol skin patch for a combined estradiol/norethisterone patch (Estracombi) for the second half of each cycle (see Figure 25)

During this phase of 12 days or so, the corpus luteum (literally 'yellow body') that comes to occupy the ruptured ovarian follicle secretes progesterone, which stabilizes the endometrium, preparing it for implantation of the fertilized ovum and thus for pregnancy. If no implantation takes place, the luteal phase normally leads to sloughing of the superficial layers of the endometrium, apparent as menstrual bleeding. Adding a progestogen to estrogen replacement therapy for 10–14 days each month has much the same effects, precipitating menstrual bleeding and thus virtually eliminating the risk of endometrial cancer. Estrogen therapy is usually continued unchanged throughout the month. It can, however, be reduced in dosage, to reflect the natural decline in secretion during the luteal phase, or be withdrawn for the last week or so of the cycle, without greatly impairing its beneficial effects on the bones, to which progestogens also contribute, though much less powerfully.

Some menopausal women taking HRT accept regular menstruation as a modest price to pay for its advantages. Many younger ones welcome it as a sign of restored sexuality, if not fertility, following a surgical or premature menopause. Older women commonly object to the continuation, and even more to the return, of the very 'curse' that

---

Table 6 Main types of progestogen-containing HRT given cyclically to protect endometrium from continuous estrogen stimulation. No combined preparations are licensed in the USA, where estrogen and progestogen have to be prescribed separately. (See Table 3 for estrogen-only preparations)

Hormone content	Typical proprietary name *	Dose
Oral preparations		
Conjugated equine estrogens Norgestrel	Prempak C	0.625, 1.25 mg 0.15 mg daily for 12 days
Estradiol valerate Norethisterone	Climagest	1 mg, 2 mg 1 mg daily for 12 days
Estradiol valerate Levonorgestrel	Cyclo-Progynova	1, 2 mg 0.25, 0.5 mg
Estradiol Estriol Norethisterone	Trisequens	2/1 or 4/1 mg 1/0.5 or 2/0.5 mg 1 mg daily for 10 days
Estradiol valerate Levonorgestrel	Nuvelle	2 mg 0.75 mg daily for 12 days
Estradiol Norethisterone	Kliofem	2 mg 1 mg
Transdermal preparation		
Estradiol Norethisterone	Estracombi (patch)	0.05 mg/24 h 0.25 mg/24 h for 14 days
Transdermal + oral preparations		
Estradiol (patch) Norethisterone (tablet)	Estrapak	0.05 mg/24 h 1 mg daily for 12 days
Estradiol (patch) Norethisterone (tablet)	Evorel-Pak	0.05 mg/24 h 1 mg daily for 12 days

* The proprietary names vary from country to country

they looked forward to being spared for the rest of their lives. The need to induce regular menstruation artificially is probably the commonest single reason for their rejecting HRT in the first place or abandoning it after a few months or years – understandably objecting that it is unnatural in itself and increasingly so in old age.

A rather different objection arises from the physical and/or psychological side-effects of progestogen therapy, which vary with the particular drug and dosage taken (Table 6) and from one woman to another. Not surprisingly, giving a progestogen to mimic the luteal phase produces much the same premenstrual effects as natural progesterone: the accumulation of fluids, which makes the body (and often the breasts in particular) feel uncomfortably bloated, sometimes accompanied by the building up of premenstrual tension, probably attributable to certain women being unusually sensitive to some or all progestogens. These undesirable effects can be minimized by trying different compounds in the lowest doses that will oppose the proliferative effect of estrogens on the endometrium.

The minimal dosage delivered by steady transdermal absorption best achieves this aim by avoiding the peak concentrations that follow single doses given by mouth (*Figure 25*). In practice, a combined skin patch (Estracombi®), delivering progestogen as well as estradiol can be applied for about 14 days each month, to mimic the luteal phase, in place of the Estraderm patch containing estradiol alone. Possible

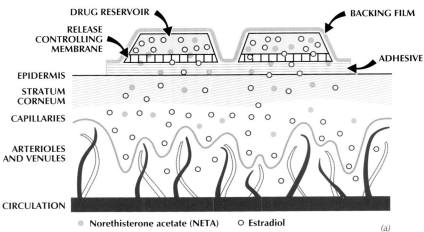

DRUG RESERVOIR   BACKING FILM
RELEASE CONTROLLING MEMBRANE   ADHESIVE
EPIDERMIS
STRATUM CORNEUM
CAPILLARIES
ARTERIOLES AND VENULES
CIRCULATION

● Norethisterone acetate (NETA)   ○ Estradiol

(a)

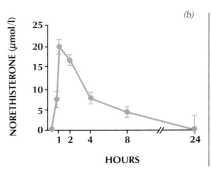

(b)

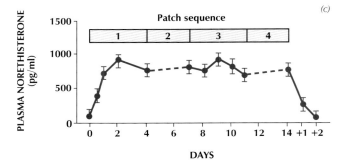

(c)

Figure 25
The Estracombi patch (a) has twin chambers but otherwise resembles the Estraderm patch illustrated in Figure 12. It releases the progestogen, norethisterone acetate (NETA) at a steady rate of 0.25 mg/24 h in addition to 50 μg of estradiol. Compared with the brief peak plasma concentrations produced by giving 1 mg NETA daily by mouth (b), controlled skin absorption from a skin patch changed twice weekly gives much more stable plasma levels over the whole 14-day course (c)

alternatives are hormone preparations that avoid the need for
induced menstruation, though they
may not completely eliminate all
irregular 'breakthrough' bleeding.
These include preparations containing a single modified sex hormone,
such as tibolone (Livial®), or continuous combined estrogen-plus-
progestogen in low dosage, but their
efficacy in combatting osteoporosis
and long-term safety have yet to be
firmly established.

**How long should HRT
be continued?**

A more critical question for every
menopausal woman seeking protection from bone loss is how long she
should continue to take HRT, of
whatever type or combination. It has
been suggested that a 10-year
course, starting at the menopause,
would strike a reasonable balance
between protecting the skeleton and
minimizing the risk of breast cancer.
Underlying this proposal is the idea
that 10 years' prevention of bone
loss should be sufficient to defer
the majority of osteoporotic fractures, which are concentrated in the
last few years of life, until the patient
has died of something else. No long-
term prospective trials comparing
HRT with other forms of preventive
therapy or with placebo have been
performed to test this plausible
notion.

For some postmenopausal
women, with a relatively high bone
mass and low rate of loss, the benefits of 10 years' HRT might well be
sufficient to justify discontinuing it

thereafter. In others, with less bone
in reserve, the accelerated loss
following withdrawal of HRT might
cancel out any benefit within 2 or 3
years. It would, of course, be impossible to identify women at risk in this
way without monitoring the bone
density. And if that were being
done, treatment might just as well
be tailored to individual needs, as it
always should be, rather than given
for any predetermined period.
Monitoring ought also to be continued if HRT is eventually withdrawn,
in case renewed bone loss requires
further preventive therapy.

**THE YOUNGER WOMAN WITH
PERSISTENT AMENORRHEA**

Many of the considerations that
influence decision-making about
postmenopausal HRT apply even
more strongly to a younger woman
– anywhere between her teens and
mid-forties – who ceases to menstruate prematurely. Hot flushes and
other characteristic symptoms may
or may not follow. But even if HRT is
not needed for symptomatic relief, it
should always be considered to
compensate for the associated lack
of estradiol if amenorrhea persists
for longer than, say, 6 months. The
alternative for a girl in her twenties
may be 50 years or more of persistent estradiol deficiency that not
only robs her of bone but also
deprives her of sexual attractiveness,
libido and cardiovascular protection.
At the same time, the induction of
regular menstruation by means of
HRT can never be more than a
second-best solution for amenorrhea
in a young woman. It cannot restore

ovulation – and therefore provides no substitute for fertility.

Surgical removal or ablation of a young woman's ovaries (or long-term suppression of their normal functioning) should be regarded as an absolute indication for starting HRT without delay (*Figure 26*). But those in whom menstruation fails to start or ceases spontaneously for no obvious reason should always be fully investigated first. Some may have a correctable cause, such as undue thinness, excessive physical exercise, or a treatable endocrine disorder. Some will have undergone a premature menopause, with irreversible though inexplicable, involution of the ovaries, as permanent as their removal, which always calls for replacement therapy. Others, including many heroin addicts, fall between these groups, in that they have potentially active ovaries but seem unlikely to adopt a lifestyle that favors their return to normal functioning. HRT may then be given to protect the bones, in the hope that estradiol secretion will take over if the natural menstrual cycle eventually resumes – perhaps when drug consumption declines and nutrition improves.

THE OLDER POSTMENOPAUSAL WOMAN

HRT can be started many years after a natural menopause. It has been shown to control bone loss when taken for the first time by older women, who may be subject to early 'senile' bone loss in addition to the continuing effects of estradiol

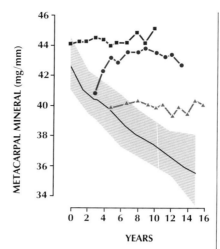

deficiency (*Figure 27*). There is no contraindication to estrogen replacement in such women on account of their age. The majority of them who still have an intact uterus may be deterred by the likelihood of erratic bleeds if they take estrogens alone or by regular menstrual loss if they add a cyclical progestogen to protect the endometrium. It may prove safe to induce bleeding at longer intervals by taking a fortnight's course of progestogen quarterly – or even annually – instead of monthly. That has yet to be established, however, and many older women might still be reluctant to resume menstruation on any terms, however infrequently.

Another drawback of starting HRT some years after the menopause is that it may have to be continued indefinitely. Otherwise, its withdrawal would precipitate a year or two of high bone turnover and accelerated

Figure 26
The reason why HRT should be started promptly in a woman of childbearing age who undergoes a surgical or premature menopause, or becomes persistently amenorrheic for any other reason. The shaded area shows the declining mineral density of metacarpal bone following bilateral oophorectomy in women receiving placebo, compared with three groups given HRT: from the time of operation (top), and starting 3 (middle), or 6 years later (bottom). Note the limited capacity of HRT to restore even 3 years' bone loss

Figure 27
The older woman, already some years past her menopause, and showing unmistakable signs of osteoporosis in this case, is no longer subject to the high rates of turnover and bone loss precipitated by recent withdrawal of estradiol. Although her persistent bone loss is still mainly caused by estrogen deficiency, and should respond well to HRT, other forms of preventive therapy may be preferred, for medical as well as personal reasons

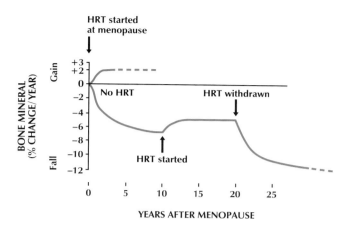

YEARS AFTER MENOPAUSE

Figure 28
Older women are prone to a 'double dip' in bone density, precipitated by renewed estrogen withdrawal, if they discontinue a course of HRT started some years after the menopause. Reduplication of the high menopausal rates of bone turnover and resorption after HRT is withdrawn may negate most of its benefits within 2 or 3 years. An older postmenopausal woman who takes HRT for the first time should therefore be prepared to continue it indefinitely or switch to another form of preventive therapy

loss at an age when senile osteoporosis might already be increasing vulnerability to fractures. This would compound the risk for an older woman who had already lost a substantial amount of bone during the earlier period of accelerated loss, following the menopause. A similar period of high turnover and accelerated loss, triggered by withdrawal of HRT as old age approaches, may be severe enough to outweigh the benefits of several years' preventive therapy. This 'double dip' in bone density (*Figure 28*) can only be avoided by continuing HRT or by substituting some other form of preventive therapy.

THE TESTOSTERONE-DEFICIENT MALE

Testosterone replacement is as much first choice for androgen-deficient men as HRT for estrogen-deficient women, with the advantage that it entails fewer serious or tiresome side-effects. Yet the proportion of such men who actually receive replacement therapy appears to be

even smaller. This must be largely due to the absence of any signs as clear-cut as amenorrhea in women, to draw attention to testosterone deficiency. This may be compounded by lack of awareness of – or unwillingness to face – a problem that hurts masculine pride, and by ignorance of the remedies available.

Like estrogens, testosterone can be given orally, transdermally or in the form of a long-acting implant. It is normally well tolerated, apart from occasional gastrointestinal or local reactions, there being no side-effects as tiresome as menstruation and few serious complications, such as increased cancer risk. Since the underlying causes of testosterone deficiency are nearly all irreversible, there is a strong case for continuing replacement therapy lifelong, provided it remains effective. Only if bone loss is not adequately controlled should it be necessary to change to an alternative (or additional) form of preventive therapy, such as a bisphosphonate or calcitonin – rather than simply withdraw testosterone and thus allow uncontrolled bone loss to recur.

THE ELDERLY PATIENT OF EITHER SEX

Although replacement therapy with appropriate sex hormones remains effective as a means of curbing bone loss in all elderly women and in testosterone-deficient men, bisphosphonates or other forms of preventive therapy usually take precedence in old people of either sex (*Figure 29*). They cannot, however, supplant

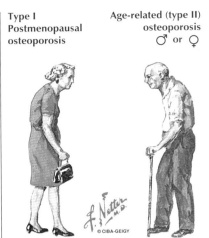

Type I Postmenopausal osteoporosis

Age-related (type II) osteoporosis ♂ or ♀

the universal need for extra calcium and vitamin D in old age, whether other forms of preventive therapy are being prescribed or not. The elderly themselves and those who care for them would also do well to heed the dietary advice of the distinguished nutritionist Dr Elsie Widdowson, who looked after her own mother to the age of 107: 'A little of what they like, and milk with everything.'

PATIENTS WITH OSTEOPOROTIC FRACTURES

Since the bone density of postmenopausal or elderly patients who have already sustained fractures will usually be close to, or below, the notional fracture threshold, their immediate need is for treatment rather than prevention of osteoporosis. Few of them get either at present, even if they sustain severe fractures in patently rarefied bone at a great age (*Figure 30*). In severely osteoporotic patients, it may be desirable to stimulate new bone

formation – so far as that is yet possible – by giving an anabolic steroid, sodium fluoride, or (for a male deficient in it) testosterone. The initial increase in bone density that takes place during the first year or two of preventive therapy with HRT, bisphosphonates or other drugs that act by inhibiting bone resorption may, however, be sufficiently effective in many cases. HRT remains the first choice following osteoporotic fractures in recently menopausal women. Once again, it must be stressed that calcium and vitamin D supplements become increasingly important with advancing age.

THE PATIENT TAKING LONG-TERM CORTICOSTEROID THERAPY

The severity of bone loss induced by corticosteroids depends on their route of administration as well as the dosage and duration of treatment. Large doses given systemically for long periods deplete the bones most. But apparently modest quantities taken regularly, even when applied locally to the skin in lotions or ointments, or inhaled from an asthma nebulizer, may cause insidious losses – which are always cumulative. What appear to be acceptably low rates of bone loss may therefore become significant if allowed to continue unchecked. This is a real danger in practice because most of the conditions for which corticosteroid therapy is indicated are chronic. The treatment controls rather than cures them, and the risk of osteoporosis will eventually be compounded by postmenopausal and/or senile bone loss.

Figure 29
The progressive bone loss that typically affects old people of both sexes will still respond to HRT in women and to testosterone among men who lack the hormone. Other forms of preventive therapy – bisphosphonates, calcitonin, fluorides or anabolic steroids – may be more appropriate and should always be accompanied by calcium and vitamin D supplements to help reduce the fracture risk (see *Figure 21*)

Figure 30
Fracture of upper shaft of left femur in a previously active woman aged 91, showing the pin, plate and fixing screws required to immobilize it surgically – an all-too typical example of treating the effects of osteoporosis while neglecting the underlying bone loss. Despite the patient's great age and the unmistakable evidence of advanced osteoporosis (complex fracture caused by minimal trauma, rarefied trabecular bone and thin cortex clearly visible on ordinary X-ray, too friable for the screws to grip), she was prescribed no specific therapy to strengthen the bones, beyond small calcium supplements of questionable value. The fracture healed on prolonged traction, enabling her to resume some activity, but only after the bones had been further weakened by over 2 months' immobility in bed

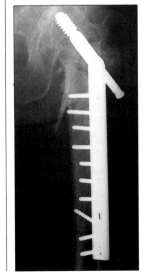

Corticosteroid-induced bone loss is hard to control because it affects bone and its remodelling in so many different ways:

■ Inhibition of the secretion of pituitary gonadotropins, leading to reduced production of estrogens in women, testosterone in men (and adrenal steroids in both sexes)

■ Reduced intestinal absorption of calcium, for which as many as nine distinct mechanisms have been identified

■ Impaired absorption and consequent deficiency of vitamin D

■ Increased PTH secretion from the parathyroid, stimulating bone resorption by the osteoclasts

■ Inhibition of osteoblast activity, decreasing bone formation

■ Increased renal excretion of calcium (which may simply be secondary to accelerated bone loss)

■ Diminished activity of growth factors that normally promote bone formation.

This diverse but incomplete list should suffice to show that corticosteroids miss few opportunities to induce bone loss, and that no single form of preventive therapy is likely to counteract them all. On the other hand, every one of the methods now available has something to offer, depending on the age and sex of the patient and on the condition requiring corticosteroid treatment. While bone loss can, therefore, be curbed in every patient taking long-term corticosteroid therapy, it can seldom be prevented altogether. Its detailed management lies beyond the scope of this book, but such an intractable problem affecting so many people unquestionably deserves earlier attention and more persistent preventive measures than it usually receives.

FULFILLING EXPECTATIONS

What can be expected from long-term preventive therapy, beyond the control of bone loss and reduction in the risk of osteoporotic fractures? Will it, for instance, add still further to the average expectation of life by preventing the many premature deaths that follow hip and other fractures? The prospects for greater longevity are surprisingly modest. It has been estimated, on the most optimistic assumptions, that 8 years' regular HRT might prolong the life of the average postmenopausal woman by anything from a couple of months to just over a year (Table 7). But increased longevity could be a questionable benefit. Not many people want to add extra months or years of poor quality to the tail-ends of their lives. Most have more realistic aspirations for their old age – to keep sufficiently active, mentally and physically, to retain their independence and to make their last years worth living. In short, they want to improve the quality of later life, not increase its quantity. That is an aim

Table 7 Will HRT prolong life? Estimated effect of at least 8 years' estrogen only or combined estrogen/progestogen replacement therapy (making optimistic and pessimistic assumptions) on life expectancy of a 50-year-old white woman

Life expectancy of woman aged 50	
No HRT	82.7 years
Estrogen only	83.7 years
Estrogen/progestogen	
optimistic	83.8 years
pessimistic	82.9 years

The modest changes anticipated in life expectancy may help to focus attention on HRT as a means of improving *quality* of life.

Relative risks of estrogen only compared with no HRT	
No HRT	1.00
Coronary heart disease	0.65
Stroke	0.95
Hip fracture	0.75
Breast cancer	1.25
(Endometrial cancer)	(8.2)

Note reductions in coronary heart disease and hip fracture, compared with increase in breast cancer. (The greatly increased risk of endometrial cancer should be eliminated by taking a cyclical progestogen.)

to which the preventive therapy of osteoporosis in general and HRT in particular can be expected to make a worthwhile contribution.

For the substantial minority of old people who would have died prematurely from a major fracture – or a stroke or heart attack, particu-larly in the case of postmenopausal women – preventive therapy offers a real prospect of adding quality as well as quantity to the last years of their lives. For the majority, the risk of chronic disability should be great-ly reduced. And for society as a whole, preventive therapy offers the only realistic prospect yet found to reduce the ever-rising financial and social burdens of caring for the disabled members of an increasingly elderly population.

These advantages can only be secured in practice if most of those at risk are sufficiently persuaded of the value of existing forms of preventive therapy to persevere with regular dosage for years on end – and that cannot be safely assumed. This ought not to be the end of the story, however. The conquest of osteoporosis, and of many of the ills of postmenopausal women, has been made possible by recent progress in developing novel methods of diagnosis, prevention and treatment. They should provide a launching pad not only for future advances in this challenging field but also for their wider implementation.

Bibliographical notes

General reviews of preventive therapy precede articles focusing on a particular drug (or group). The aim is to present the well-informed views of specialists experienced in the management of osteoporosis, as being of more practical value to the reader than clinical trial reports as such. The first group of references presents an overall picture [Cooper J.C. et al. (1994), Osteoporosis: recent advances in pathogenesis and treatment, Q. J. Med., **87**, 203–9; Kanis, J.A. (1993), What constitutes evidence of drug efficacy in osteoporosis? Drugs Aging, **3**, 391–9; Patel S. et al. (1993), Drugs used in the treatment of metabolic bone disease; clinical pharmacology and therapeutic use, Drugs, **46**, 594–617; Piziak V.K. (1994), Update in osteoporosis, Compr. Ther., **20**, 336–41; Cormier C. (1993), Epidemiology, diagnosis and treatment of osteoporosis, Curr. Opin. Rheumatol., **6**, 329–35; Harris S.T. (1993), Osteoporosis: pharmacologic treatment strategies, Adv. Intern. Med., **38**, 303–21; Recker R.R. (1993), Clinical Review 41, J. Clin. Endocrinol. Metab., **76**, 14–16; Choice of drugs for postmenopausal osteoporosis (1992), Med. Lett. Drugs Ther., **34**, 101–2; Evantash E.G. et al. (1994), Prevention and treatment of osteoporosis, Compr. Ther., **20**, 253–6].

The following references are grouped by drug type, starting with estrogens/HRT [Filer W.D. et al. (1994), Transdermal estrogen and prevention of osteoporosis, Am. Fam. Physician, **49**, 1639–44; Lindsay R. (1993), Hormone replacement therapy for prevention and treatment of osteoporosis, Am. J. Med., **95 suppl. 5A**, 37S–39S; Barlow D.H. (1993), HRT and osteoporosis, Baillieres Clin. Rheumatol., **7**, 535–48; De Cherney A. (1993), Physiologic and pharmacologic effects of estrogen and progestins on bone, J. Reprod. Med., **38 suppl. 12**, 1007–14; Ettinger B. (1993), Use of low-dose 17-beta estradiol for the prevention of osteoporosis, Clin. Ther., **15**, 950–62; te Velde E.R. et al. (1994), Hormonal treatment for the climacteric: alleviation of symptoms and prevention of postmenopausal disease, Lancet, **343**, 654–8; Lindsay R. (1993), Criteria for successful estrogen therapy in osteoporosis, Osteoporos. Int., **3 suppl. 2**, 9–13; Lindsay R. et al. (1993), Estrogen: effects and actions in osteoporosis, Osteoporos. Int., **3 suppl. 1**, 150–2; Yun S. et al. (1993), Medroxyprogesterone in osteoporosis, Ann. Pharmacother., **27**, 448–9; Compston J.E. (1992), HRT and osteoporosis, Br. Med. Bull., **48**, 309–44; Balfour J.A. et al. (1992), Transdermal estradiol. A review of its pharmacological profile and therapeutic potential in the prevention of postmenopausal osteoporosis, Drugs Aging, **2**, 487–507; Christiansen C. (1993), Prevention and treatment of osteoporosis with hormone replacement therapy, Int. J. Fertil. Menopausal Stud., **38 suppl. 1**, 45–54]. One paper particularly considers alternatives to HRT in prevention and treatment [Marsh M.S. et al. (1993), Baillieres Clin. Rheumatol., **7**, 549–60].

The risk of breast cancer in patients taking long-term HRT is comprehensively reviewed in a recent book [Hormone Replacement Therapy and Breast Cancer Risk, Mann R.D. (ed.), Parthenon Publishing Group, Carnforth, 1992] and article [Barrett-Connor E. (1994), Postmenopausal estrogen and the risk of breast cancer, Ann. Epidemiol., **4**, 177–80, and comment: 255–6]. The question remains controversial, however [Colditz G. A. *et al.* (1995), The use of estrogens and progestins and the risk of breast cancer in postmenopausal women, *N. Engl. J. Med.*, **332**, 1589–93; Stanford J. L. *et al.* (1995), Combined estrogen and progestin hormone replacement therapy in relation to risk of breast cancer in middle-aged women, *JAMA*, **274**, 137–42].

Recent bisphosphonate references cover some new compounds as well as those already available [Papapoulos S.E. (1993), Role of bisphosphonates in the prevention and treatment of osteoporosis, *Am. J. Med.*, **95 suppl. 5A**, 48S–52S; Ott S.M. (1993), Clinical effects of bisphosphonates in involutional osteoporosis, *J. Bone Min. Res.*, **8 Suppl. 2**, S597–606; Licata, A.A. (1993), From bathtub ring to osteoporosis: a clinical review of the bisphosphonates, *Cleve. Clin. J. Med.*, **60**, 284–90; Fleisch H. (1993), New bisphosphonates in osteoporosis, *Osteoporos. Int.*, **3 suppl. 2**, S15–22; Kanis J.A. *et al.* (1993), Rationale for the use of clodronate in osteoporosis, *Osteoporos. Int.*, **3 suppl. 2**, S23–8; Sørensen O.H. *et al.* (1993), Bisphosphonates and osteoporosis, *Osteoporos. Int.*, **3 suppl. 1**, 223–5; Reginster J.Y. (1992), Oral tiludronate, pharmacological properties and potential usefulness in Paget's disease of bone and osteoporosis, *Bone*, **13**, 351–4; Stone M. (1993), Didronel PMO, *Br. J. Hosp. Med.*, **49**, 275–7; Bijvoet O.L. *et al.* (1993), Bisphosphonates in osteoporosis? *Osteoporos. Int.*, **3 suppl. 1**, 230–6; Calcitonin is the subject of relatively few reports [Reginster J.Y. (1993), Calcitonin for prevention and treatment of osteoporosis, *Am. J. Med.*, **95 suppl. 5A**, 44S–47S; Wallach S. (1992), The role of calcitonin treatment in postmenopausal osteoporosis, *Orthop. Rev.*, **21**, 1034–42 and 1130–1; Gennari C. *et al.* (1993), Long-term treatment with calcitonin in osteoporosis, *Horm. Metab. Res.*, **25**, 484–5].

Fluoride continues to attract interest, as the main means of promoting bone formation [Kanis, J.A. (1993), Treatment of symptomatic osteoporosis with fluoride, *Am. J. Med.*, **95 suppl. 5A**, 53S-61S; Dequeker J. *et al.* (1993), Fluor in the treatment of osteoporosis. An overview of 30 years clinical research, *Schweiz. Med. Wochenschr.*, **123**, 2228–34; Boivin G. *et al.* (1993), Fluoride and osteoporosis, *World Rev. Nutr. Diet*, **73**, 80–103; Kleerekoper M. *et al.* (1993), Sodium fluoride therapy of postmenopausal osteoporosis, *Endocr. Rev.*, **14**, 312–3] and the search for alternative means of stimulating bone formation continues [Riggs B.L. (1993), Formation-stimulating regimens other than sodium fluoride, *Am. J. Med.*, **95 suppl. 5A**, 62S–68S].

The benefits of calcium supplements, vitamin D, diet and exercise are examined in several papers [Prince R. (1993), The calcium controversy revisited: implications of new data, *Med. J. Aust.*, **159**, 404–7; Harward M.P. (1993), Nutritive therapies for osteoporosis. The role of calcium, *Med. Clin. North Am.*, **77**, 889–98; Sambrook P. (1992), Calcitriol and postmenopausal osteoporosis, *Med. J. Aust.*, **157**, 364–6; Vargo M.M. *et al.* (1993), Exercise strategies for osteoporosis, *Bull. Rheum. Dis.*, **42**, 6–9; Ernst E. (1994), Can exercise prevent postmenopausal osteoporosis? *Br. J. Sports Med.*, **28**, 5–6].

Two recent papers focus on the major challenge of treatment for osteoporosis in old age [Rubin C.D. (1993), Osteoporosis: considerations in evaluating and managing the older patient, *Tex. Med.*, **10**, 67–74; Seymour D.G. *et al.* (1994), Prospects for treating osteoporosis in older people, *J. R. Soc. Med.*, **87 suppl. 23**, 26–30].

Chapter 7:
Follow-up and future prospects

IMPROVING THE PROGNOSIS

For all the diagnostic and therapeutic progress made in recent years, osteoporosis is far from conquered. Clinical trials apart, no convincing overall reduction in osteoporotic fractures has yet been reported among the members of any high-risk population anywhere in the world. Nowhere are the preventive measures now available being applied widely enough, or continued long enough, for that desirable aim even to be in prospect. The importance of building up the bone mass in children and adolescents has scarcely begun to be recognized – and scant attention is being paid to its maintenance later in life. Accelerated bone loss continues unabated in the great majority of postmenopausal women and old people, and in the growing number of younger adults now identifiably at risk, who could be receiving preventive therapy, but are not. Individually, the prognosis has yet to be improved in more than a trifling minority, consisting chiefly of the few women taking long-term HRT as a preventive measure and the small numbers of either sex receiving belated treatment for established osteoporosis. Collectively, the outlook must still be deteriorating wherever people are living longer and the numerous other causes of bone loss remain unchecked.

Even among the minority of those at risk who are fortunate enough to start preventive therapy in good time, it is uncertain how much the prognosis may be improved – or for how long. Not all of them will have bone densities that are already low or falling unduly fast. They would obviously benefit most, but there is no reliable way to identify them in advance without much wider use of densitometry to screen the bones of all those potentially at risk. Much of today's depressingly small amount of preventive prescribing therefore goes to patients selected more haphazardly. They may or may not be at high risk – or adequately investigated, treated or followed-up.

HIT AND MISS PRESCRIBING

Most postmenopausal women taking long-term HRT start it to relieve hot flushes and other acute symptoms of estrogen withdrawal, but continue for quite different reasons: some for its beneficial effects on their general health, wellbeing or libido, others for the sake of their bones. Many of them do so, whether at their own request or on medical advice, without having their bone density measured initially or monitored to assess their response to HRT or to its eventual withdrawal. That they are all estradiol deficient is not, of course, in question – and a sound case can be made for hormone replacement on that account alone. But not all estradiol-deficient women are equally prone to osteoporosis. Their rates of bone loss vary widely, both between individuals and from time to time. Barely half of those who live into old age sustain one or more osteoporotic fractures by their 80th birthday. Although many of them would have been identifiable by their low bone density as much as 25 years earlier, not nearly enough women undergo densito-metry soon after the menopause for those already at high risk to have much chance of being identified at that crucial stage. Prescribing of long-term HRT as preventive therapy is therefore largely hit-and-miss.

The case for investigation is especially strong among the growing number of amenorrheic younger women who become estradiol-deficient early in what would normally be their childbearing years, sometimes starting as early as their late teens. Amenorrhea makes them all quite readily identifiable, but the risk of their becoming prematurely osteoporotic is obviously greatest if the condition is irreversible. These unfortunate young women face several decades of bone loss before they reach middle age. It is vital that they should be distinguished from the majority, including about 50%

of competitive athletes and many anorexia sufferers, whose amenor-rhea and estrogen deficiency are usually self-correcting when they gain weight by putting on sufficient body fat. This is normally enough to restore the balance of bone remodelling, even if it does not enable them to regain all the bone already lost. Yet the vital distinction between permanent and reversible amenorrhea tends to be neglected for months or years, and sometimes indefinitely, before its causes are investigated. Even when it is known to be irreversible in a young woman, following confirmation of a premature menopause, or its induction by medical or surgical means, she may not have her bone density measured or the resulting hormone loss replaced.

The chances of densitometry being performed or preventive therapy prescribed appear to be poorer still among other groups identifiably at risk. Reprehensibly few of the many patients, young or old of either sex, who are now taking long-term corticosteroids have had either the risk of osteoporosis assessed by monitoring the bone density or the need for preventive therapy seriously considered by the doctors prescribing them. The position is little better among men who are found to be testosterone-deficient. The diagnosis of this near-symptomless condition is commonly missed or delayed. If eventually made, it may already have been responsible for years of bone loss. Yet neither the investigation of the minority who come to diagnostic light nor their treatment with testosterone will necessarily be directed to the long-term prevention of osteoporosis or accompanied by monitoring of the bone density.

Most of the numerous patients who sustain fractures in osteoporotic bones also continue to escape the diagnostic net, even though the great majority are patently postmenopausal or elderly. The small proportion of them now taking preventive therapy of any kind must be outnumbered tens of times over by the countless fracture patients whose low bone densities and persistently high rates of bone loss still go unchecked – in both senses. The overall prognosis can hardly be expected to improve so long as preventive therapy continues to be poorly aimed at so few of its prospective targets.

PREVENTION IN PRACTICE

Poor targeting of preventive therapy on those at high risk is just one of many reasons why it may be less effective in practice than the favorable results of clinical trials might suggest. Lack of monitoring in many non-trial patients masks the discrepancy, which can arise from various sources. They all have their roots in the contrast between the highly disciplined conduct of controlled trials and the more haphazard conditions that inevitably surround prescribing in everyday practice. Their aims are, after all, fundamentally different.

Clinical trials are invariably designed to answer specific questions, usually concerned with evaluating the efficacy and safety of one form of drug treatment, compared with others or with placebo. They always seek to do so under precisely defined conditions, in particular types of patient satisfying strict inclusion and exclusion criteria. When prescribing for individual patients, by contrast, clinicians have to do their best for every one of them in the prevailing circumstances, however unfavorable. The strict criteria for entry to a trial could not be imposed in practice without excluding many patients from much-needed treatment. The regular administration of a set drug in standardized dosage, necessary for trial purposes, can never be optimal for every individual. Some may need a different drug, higher dosage or additional measures to produce a satisfactory response, others a lower dose or an alternative drug to minimize side-effects or avoid conflict with another disorder or its treatment. Some trial conditions are too restrictive or the frequency of check-ups too intrusive for the patient, or too time-consuming for the doctor, to be acceptable in practice. Expectations of benefit may also differ radically.

Trials designed to assess the merits of preventive therapy usually do so by measuring its effect on bone density over a conveniently short period. The maintenance or modest enhancement of density for a year or two, compared with placebo-treated controls who are still losing bone, is generally considered sufficient to demonstrate a drug's capacity to prevent osteoporosis. But that is by no means the same thing as its lifelong prevention. Relatively few trials have been based on long-term reduction in fracture rates, most of them confined to the vertebral bodies of recently menopausal women. Certainly, no controlled trial has yet been continued for long enough to demonstrate what patients and doctors considering the pros and cons of preventive therapy most need to know: whether it will reduce the lifetime risk of osteoporotic fractures and disabilities, including the life-threatening hip fractures of old age. The extent to which that desirable aim may be attainable in practice, therefore, remains uncertain.

Bone loss may not be curbed effectively enough to minimize the long-term risk of fractures, if the preventive therapy prescribed is not well-suited to the patient, if its dosage is too low, the period of treatment too short, or the response inadequate in particular bones or the skeleton as a whole. The patient may take it irregularly, or abandon it prematurely, perhaps without telling the doctor, through side-effects (or fear of them), for lack of motivation to continue treatment for years on end, or simply from forgetfulness, especially in the elderly whose need is often greatest. Even if preventive therapy is eventually discontinued on medical advice, the increased bone loss that invariably follows

may be overlooked. Such pitfalls attract little attention because the bone loss that follows withdrawal of preventive therapy is symptomless until a fracture occurs, often too long afterwards for the link between cause and effect to be apparent. This sequence of events must be commonplace in practice but usually goes undetected for lack of bone monitoring. Yet there is little margin for such errors and omissions.

Even if all these diagnostic, therapeutic and behavioral pitfalls could be avoided, the biological response to a particular drug and dosage would still vary over quite a broad range, maintaining the bone density well above the notional fracture threshold in some patients but failing to do so in others. The biological response to withdrawal of preventive therapy also varies, making the rate and duration of subsequent bone loss unpredictable. Neither an unusually poor response nor an exceptionally severe recurrence will be apparent, unless the bone density is monitored both during and after treatment. Many a slip separates prescribing from effective prevention, which always has to contend with the persistent forces that are constantly awaiting their chance to promote accelerated bone loss.

ADVERSE (HUMAN) INFLUENCES STILL AT WORK

There can be little doubt that the 20th century growth in osteoporosis is still continuing, since most of its recognized causes are still at work and tending to increase rather than decline. There is no reason to suppose that this growth owes anything to genetic changes. Its causes lie almost exclusively in the cumulative effects on *normal* bone of the wide range of human activities discussed in previous chapters. Only when the factors promoting bone loss are considered as a whole does it become apparent how numerous they are, how insidiously they act, how much they have increased in recent years, and what a large proportion of that increase is man-made.

The lesson for the future is clear. More effective prevention of osteoporosis calls for constant vigilance to spot any increase in the factors known to cause osteo-porosis, and any novel ones that might do so, before they have done too much damage. Two examples of the latter have recently come under suspicion, both affecting men, for a change. Cannabis smoking tends to reduce blood levels of testosterone, sometimes quite markedly. And reports of a near-50% fall in the sperm counts of European men over the past half-century suggest that this could have been accompanied by a decline in testosterone secretion, and consequently in bone density, over the same period. In either case, some middle-aged and elderly men could now have weaker bones more prone to osteoporotic fractures than those of previous generations.

Such speculation aside, the natural life history of adult bone is tilted towards loss in both sexes. Once the needs of growth and reproduction have been served, remodelling is, therefore, more easily pushed to greater losses than brought back into balance. The various contributory causes of osteoporosis, which all act by exaggerating this biological trait, are not effectively resisted by countervailing influences. Indeed, it is only possible to identify three of any importance: the 75-year-old discovery that rickets and osteomalacia could be prevented by vitamin D and calcium, and the comparatively recent introduction of the contraceptive pill and of HRT and other forms of preventive therapy for osteoporosis itself. Against that, the various human activities that have greatly increased the problem of osteoporosis in western industrialized peoples must now be insidiously promoting bone loss in numerous other societies around the world – east and west, developing and underdeveloped. Wherever life expectancy is rising alongside the spread of industrialization and westernization, including the advent of modern medicine, the largely unrecognized problem of osteoporosis must also be growing.

THE GLOBAL PERSPECTIVE

About two-thirds of the old people who have ever lived on earth are estimated to be alive today, and nearly two-thirds of them are postmenopausal women. The growing burdens that hip and other fractures already impose on many of them, on their families, on local communities, on health and social services and thus on everybody's taxes, have yet to be relieved in any part of the world. These seem certain to become worldwide problems – with many local variations.

In the UK, one person in every five is now an old-age pensioner, and that unprecedented proportion will have risen to one in four by quite early in the next century. There will then be little more than one full-time worker to support each pensioner, even if unemployment is low. The burdens that osteoporosis and the many other ills of old age impose on each worker/taxpayer are bound to follow this pattern in all industrialized countries and may rise further. Many of the people retiring in the next few decades will be entering old age with bones predictably weaker than those of recent generations, and therefore more prone to fractures and chronic disability.

The western world, which showed the way to increased longevity and unwittingly increased the risk of osteoporosis, now has the opportunity to counter the adverse influences on bone density – at a price. But the problem is no longer confined to the west. Many developing countries already have unprecedented numbers living for longer than ever before and increasingly subject to many of the adverse influences known to

promote bone loss. Few of these countries will be able to give any priority to densitometry or to afford long-term preventive therapy on the necessary scale. Despite their contemporary problems, they have nevertheless been able to cut some corners in health care – thanks to lessons learned earlier in Europe and North America.

As the industrial revolution of the eighteenth and nineteenth centuries spread from Britain to western Europe and then to the USA, it was followed by several generations of sharply diminished life expectancy as countless country people migrated to overcrowded, insanitary urban slums where disease flourished alongside the new industries and many died prematurely. Among infections, vitamin deficiencies and other disorders that had been rare in the country, rickets and osteomalacia became commonplace among the new towndwellers, cut off both from plentiful supplies of calcium and vitamin D in milk and from the sunlight to synthesize the latter for themselves. They were as much man-made diseases of their time as osteoporosis is today. Yet there are important differences between the industrial urbanization of the past and the corresponding movements taking place in developing countries today.

Many of the public health lessons were learned, of necessity, the first time round. If they had not been – if the importance of clean water and hygienic sewage disposal were not now understood, if vaccines, antibiotics and insecticides had not been developed to bring infectious diseases under control, if vitamins had not been discovered – the hundreds of millions of erstwhile country people who have crowded into the shanty towns and slums of Third-world cities in the past 50 years would have led brief lives, cut short by disease. Infant mortality would have soared way above its present high levels, and periodic epidemics, particularly of plague, cholera and typhus, would have swept millions to early deaths. The average expectation of life, at birth, could well have fallen below the mid-teens, as it did in early-nineteenth century London. But that has not happened at all widely in even the poorest of today's developing countries. Except sporadically, as a result of wars and natural disasters, the overcrowded populations of Third-world cities are not being decimated by disease. Most of them are still enlarging, not only because the birth rate is high and more country people keep arriving, but because many of their inhabitants are living longer.

Industrialization and urbanization in developing countries bring many social and medical problems in their wake, but they are not being accompanied by the severe falls in life expectancy – or even by rickets and osteomalacia on anything like the scale once commonplace in European and North American cities. Instead, they are in the main leading directly, without an intervening dip, to growing longevity.

The average life expectancy at birth, for developing countries as a whole, is estimated to have risen by more than 50%, from 40 to 63 years, since the mid-1950s. At that time, most women died well before reaching menopausal age. Today, unprecedented numbers spend 10 years or more in the postmenopausal state, and many men as well as women are living into old age – increasingly prone to degenerative diseases, including osteoporosis.

THE RISING RISK

This problem is beginning to be recognized among the predominantly light-boned people of Japan, the acknowledged leader of late-twentieth century industrialization. Their already high life expectancy is thought to be rising faster than anywhere else and now appears to be the highest on earth. The resulting increase in osteoporotic fractures is attracting some preventive attention, but the main remedies so far adopted – calcium supplements and the largely self-selected use of HRT – are being taken by relatively few well-motivated postmenopausal women, as in the west. It is seldom selectively targeted on high-risk individuals. Total consumption of HRT still appears to be low, suggesting that it is not being taken nearly widely enough, and quite probably not in adequate dosage or for long enough, to reduce overall fracture rates.

Among other Asian populations known to be susceptible, notably the Chinese with their intolerance to milk and low consumption, in south-east Asia, and in India, where the average life expectancy has also been rising dramatically in recent decades, osteoporosis receives little attention. Priority is understandably given to more pressing health problems. Yet bone loss cannot be safely ignored or considered in isolation. Growing numbers of elderly people, for whom there are reasonably reliable population statistics from most countries, must result in more osteoporotic fractures, which are not yet being accurately counted. Their emergency treatment, together with any aftercare of the disabilities that result, will inevitably divert scarce medical resources away from life-threatening infections, malnutrition, maternity and child welfare services, AIDS prevention, and other major priorities. Health authorities everywhere face similar dilemmas, arising from the need to satisfy almost limitless demand from strictly limited resources.

However much the details differ from one part of the world to another, similar population movements and age trends are accompanying industrialization and urbanization in many parts of Asia, in much of the former Soviet bloc, and in Central and South America. Rising life expectancy and the adoption of more western lifestyles, coupled with the European or Oriental origins of many of their peoples must be making them increasingly susceptible to osteoporosis. To a lesser degree, the same applies in Africa and among black people of African origin, notably in the USA and Caribbean. Although their bones are genetically more robust, fractures still become more common after the menopause and rise further in old age. Black people are not immune to osteoporotic bone loss or its effects, just less susceptible. Everywhere, the need to prevent osteoporosis will continue to grow as more people live longer. But when will that need be recognized? How widely, and how effectively, can a response be made? The answers depend as much on improving delivery of existing methods to those in need, as on further technical advances.

WHAT CAN BE DONE NOW

For most people at risk – and for too many of their doctors – it is as if recent advances in the understanding, diagnosis and preventive therapy of osteoporosis had never been made. The most pressing measures that could be taken without more ado are therefore to increase public and professional awareness of osteoporosis, with the aim of focusing attention on the four key areas repeatedly stressed here but still neglected in practice: *building up strong bones in youth, identifying adults at high risk, offering them preventive therapy, and monitoring the response.*

The results of different schemes would also need to be collated and published, not simply to establish which were the most cost-effective but also to make the information widely known. Only if large numbers of doctors as well as parents and prospective patients become convinced of the value of lifelong prevention can much progress be expected. Even in western countries where the risk of osteoporosis is greatest and the necessary remedies could be most readily afforded, there has been little discussion about who should provide medical care on the scale required – general practitioners backed by open access to hospital densitometry facilities? – specialists in gynecology, rheumatology, general medicine, or orthopedics? – or the slowly growing number of menopause clinics?

As these are all fully occupied if not overburdened at present, it is far from clear where the necessary expertise could be found, bearing in mind the dearth of clinical specialists in osteoporosis as such and the huge numbers at risk. A network of osteoporosis clinics, with specially trained staff and equipped with densitometry facilities, would almost certainly be required to cope with the workload. But health authorities would probably not be prepared to establish them without clear evidence both of the need and of their cost effectiveness. Neither is readily available at present. Nor has public or professional opinion yet exerted the campaigning pressure that gave priority to cervical smears and breast screening – before their preventive value had been firmly established.

At best, the prevention of osteoporosis with the means available today cannot be more than an extended holding operation. It may well continue to be limited to a minority of those at risk who are determined to take long-term preventive therapy. For those who fail to persevere, it could soon turn out to be a losing struggle that fails to reduce the risk of fracture. What more has the future to offer? Are there realistic prospects of osteoporosis being conquered more decisively, by simpler and cheaper means, which could be made more readily available to the great majority of those at risk?

WHAT MAY BECOME POSSIBLE IN THE FUTURE

Osteoporosis differs from degenerative conditions which follow a remorseless downwards course. Unlike them, it is potentially reversible, because osteoporotic bone continues to be remodelled, still has the capacity to regenerate and repair itself following fractures, and retains its sensitivity to circumstance, both adverse and favorable. All these related processes provide openings for their own modification which are virtually unique to bone. This makes the prevention of osteoporosis not merely possible but practicable – and eminently worthwhile.

The future therefore beckons beguilingly – promising numerous technical advances in the prevention and treatment of osteoporosis. Compared with present methods, the possibilities are far more diverse in their scope and likely to be more selective, more potent and perhaps potentially more hazardous in some of their effects. All manner of novel possibilities will be opened up as the basic mechanisms of biology, the role of genetics in the synthesis and mineralization of normal bone, and its susceptibility to environmental factors, both internal and external, come to be better understood. But progress on the anticipated scale is also likely to contain traps for the unwary. Doctors and patients alike could easily be lured into the uncritical adoption of deceptively attractive technical 'solutions', which would not necessarily remedy the problems they were supposed to solve and might well create some unexpected new ones. Caution may be particularly appropriate here, bearing in mind that most of the twentieth-century increase in osteoporosis has arisen unexpectedly from adopting attractive solutions to other problems.

The medicine of the future must learn to choose critically and thriftily from the preventive and therapeutic wonders that science will increasingly have on offer. The last few decades have demonstrated the need to exercise unaccustomed judgements as technical barriers have fallen. Some of the medical problems created by scientific progress are mainly ethical, notably in such fields as setting limits to genetic engineering in man or pathogenic micro-organisms,

defining the moment of death in an injured organ donor, and deciding when a brain-dead patient should have the life-support systems switched off. Setting limits to the exploitation of 'therapeutically' aborted fetuses is arguably the trickiest of all, when harsh choices have to be made between incineration on one hand and the unique value of this source of human tissues for transplantation, for research into infertility and embryonic development, and for obtaining ova from female fetuses for 'test-tube' fertilization and uterine implantation into women unable to conceive naturally. In these and other instances, the diagnostic, prophylactic and therapeutic advances thrown up by science have economic as well as ethical dimensions. If a new, potentially life-preserving technique is inordinately expensive, and only available to a minority of patients, how should these patients be selected and on what grounds?

Questions of affordability and cost-effectiveness are becoming inextricably bound up with medical ethics in a world where palliative treatment of a thus-far incurable condition like AIDS can run to tens of thousands of pounds per patient-year. The cost of preventing osteoporosis would be relatively low per head but many times higher than the total currently spent on AIDS because the numbers at risk from bone loss are vastly greater. Which should take precedence? For what reasons? And who is to decide? Are the elderly more expendable than the young? Should non-smokers take therapeutic precedence over smokers, as has recently been suggested? The need to find answers to such imponderable questions is already pressing in many fields of medicine. Osteoporosis may join them as people become increasingly aware that it is common, disabling, life-threatening, costly – and preventable. The technical developments forecast in the remainder of this chapter will therefore need to be evaluated, not in research studies and clinical trials alone, but for their cost-effectiveness under real-life conditions and in relation to the many competing and ever-increasing demands on limited health-care resources.

COMBATTING THE CAUSES

The diverse causes of osteoporosis provide an obvious approach, not yet fully exploited, to improved methods of prevention. Some, such as dietary calcium deficiency, can be corrected as such; others, like lack of estradiol or testosterone, can be compensated for by replacement therapy. Future attention could turn to more radical solutions, taking numerous different forms. The therapeutic properties of corticosteroid drugs, for instance, cannot yet be separated from their adverse effects on calcium absorption and bone remodelling, but future research may find a way. Equally, there is no practical means of enhancing calcium absorption at present, apart from taking many times more by mouth (whether in

the diet or as supplements) than the body needs, and continuing to do so indefinitely. Yet there must be ways of promoting absorption of dietary calcium, perhaps by mimicking, or improving on, the mechanisms by which the body normally does so in infancy and adolescence.

Amenorrhea and estradiol deficiency may not be as inseparably associated with low body weight in young women as they appear to be, because there is quite wide individual variation. This is also true of bone loss in the elderly, which may not be a wholly inevitable consequence of aging. Ways might be found to break such links if their mechanisms were better understood. Many of the causes of osteoporosis could prove less intractable than they now seem, once they were taken seriously enough to stimulate closer study of their mechanisms, as has already been happening in the search for improved methods of preventing postmenopausal bone loss.

IMPROVING HRT

The most obvious need in postmenopausal women is for simpler, more sophisticated ways of preventing osteoporosis that do not entail years of regular medication and artificially prolonged menstruation. For all the proven efficacy of HRT, and the near restoration of premenopausal conditions when estradiol is given transdermally, present methods still fall short of the ideal. It might, for example, be possible to develop a modified estrogen-like steroid which acted more selectively in protecting the bones and cardiovascular system without stimulating the endometrium. That should be welcomed by many women, because it would avoid the need both for cyclical progestogen and for monthly bleeds. Their compliance might be further improved by long-acting hormone (or other) therapy that only needed to be taken intermittently, as a short course or, best of all, in a single dose, to give long-term protection from bone loss.

Obviating the need to take regular doses for years on end should also reduce side-effects and, of course, greatly lower the cost of HRT. This might be achieved by a sophisticated hormone implant releasing a consistently metered dosage over months or years. Alternatively, a way might be found to implant ovarian tissue containing potentially active follicular cells, perhaps cultured from a small biopsy of the patient's own ovaries taken well before the menopause (or at the time of their surgical removal). Such an implant would avoid the need for hormone treatment if it proved capable of secreting sufficient quantities of estradiol cyclically, under normal pituitary control, and perhaps for the rest of the patient's life. It would, however, induce regular menstruation in women with an intact uterus, but ablation of the endometrial lining already offers a simpler alternative to hysterectomy for solving that problem.

Future developments could go further. Women may not always be content with the undemanding yardstick that HRT should not increase the high existing risk of breast or uterine cancer. A truly ideal form of replacement therapy would not only correct estradiol deficiency, thus preventing osteoporosis and cardiovascular disease, but reduce or even eliminate the 'normal' cancer risks. Manipulation of the extraordinarily versatile steroid molecule might just produce a modified sex hormone, or a combination of two or more, with all these desirable actions, possibly in the form of a long-acting implant.

Similarly, a long-acting preparation of modified testosterone might be capable of maintaining the bone density, without some of it being metabolized into dihydrotestosterone, which seems to be responsible for prostatic enlargement in older men. It is also conceivable that the high 'normal' risk of prostatic cancer could also be reduced in some such way. If compliance with improved forms of HRT could be assured in both sexes, and their control of bone loss were sufficiently consistent, it might no longer be necessary to monitor the individual response – any more than each child needs to be tested for antibodies to measles or diphtheria after being vaccinated against them.

However much HRT may be improved in the future, it could only be effective in women or men lacking the estradiol or testosterone that would normally maintain the strength of their bones. Alternative means would, therefore, be required to balance the remodelling processes, and promote calcium absorption, in all other patients. This might be achieved by refining the existing forms of preventive therapy or by mimicking the actions of the local mediators that normally control osteoclast and osteoblast function.

STIMULATING BONE FORMATION ...

An improved means of promoting new bone formation, more potent than those currently available and suitable for the preventive therapy of senile osteoporosis as well as the treatment of advanced disease, has already been identified as an aim of future research. If an anabolic steroid or other compound could be developed which acted as a powerful stimulant of osteoblastic activity, the bone already lost by a severely osteoporotic patient of either sex could be replaced to an unprecedented extent. Any such drug would, however, be almost certain to have the inherent limitation of being unable to reunite ruptured trabeculae. The gaps between their broken stumps could not be bridged by cells confined to working on bone surfaces, as osteoblasts are, unless new bone formation could somehow be concentrated at their tips, enabling them to grow outwards towards each other. Even this seemingly remote possibility may not be beyond the bounds of biological ingenuity, though other methods

(discussed below) seem more likely to solve the problem. In any event, greater power to stimulate bone formation would have to be accompanied by correspondingly greater care in its use.

... WITHIN LIMITS

Feedback control of remodelling normally prevents new bone formation in adults from exceeding the rate of resorption. Nature has played safe by tilting the overall balance slightly towards loss. Even in pathological conditions, it is exceedingly rare for excessive bone to build up in human or other animal skeletons. During the long course of evolution, weightier bones must have been tried and found wanting. In the harsh world of natural selection, maintaining a stronger but more cumbersome skeleton presumably made excessive dietary and metabolic demands without conferring any advantage over lighter-boned, more agile rivals. Therapeutic enthusiasm for more potent drugs to stimulate bone formation would have to be tempered with caution.

If science devises more satisfactory means than anabolic steroids or fluoride salts to overrule nature's controls and generate new bone of normal structure and strength, it would also be necessary to monitor its rate of formation and ensure that the bone mass was kept within physiological bounds. Otherwise, some elderly patients might find themselves saddled with skeletons which not only imposed excessive dietary and metabolic demands but also overburdened their waning muscle power. Such fracture-proofing of the aging skeleton as may be possible would do better to emulate nature than risk driving it to such excesses. The basic design of human and other animal bones, in which structure and function are always so admirably matched, needs to be retained as far as possible in old age, not artificially distorted. This might be achieved by exploring ways of mimicking the positive effects of puberty on both bone mass and calcium absorption. In both sexes, these benefits seem to result from the combined action of the relevant sex hormones, together with growth hormone, and possibly other factors, on immature adolescent bones (which may be unusually sensitive to their effects). It might become possible to produce similar changes in mature, even elderly, bones.

LOCAL REINFORCEMENT?

It may not always be necessary to think in terms of general measures to protect and strengthen the entire skeleton. A strong case can be made for *local* strengthening of the bones most susceptible to serious fractures, notably the vertebral bodies and femoral neck. This might be done in various ways. The exploitation of the local physiological response to weight-bearing exertion must be the simplest. Exercises specifically designed to stress the lumbar spine, the femoral neck and forearm bones should help to limit loss from these

critical areas – and the benefit could no doubt be intensified by giving HRT or some other form of systemic therapy at the same time. More fundamental approaches may become possible as more is learned about the physiological mechanisms by which physical stress (or lack of it) influences remodelling. Distortion of hydroxyapatite crystals is thought to produce a local piezo-electric effect to which the osteocytes appear to respond by stimulating osteoblastic formation of new bone. This mechanism could perhaps be mimicked or enhanced by inducing similar electrical changes in bones at high risk, or by developing synthetic chemical mediators resembling those that normally stimulate local osteoblastic activity.

Other preventive and/or therapeutic possibilities arise from the fact that certain bones (or parts of them) are prone to unusually high rates of loss. They must be responding to local mechanisms or localized sensitivity to systemic influences. Once the mediators concerned were identified, ways could probably be found to block their action – and thus prevent the accelerated bone loss they would otherwise cause. Alternatively, the presence of specific mediators (or their receptors) at particular sites might enable them to be used as targets for systemic treatment to home in on – and thus act locally where its effect was most needed.

Given sufficient biochemical and microbiological ingenuity, an anabolic steroid or bisphosphonate might be developed in the form of a 'pro-drug'. Ideally, this would be inert when taken by mouth and remain so in the rest of the body, until activated locally by specific enzymes or transmitters present only (or mainly) in the target tissue. Or such a pro-drug could be activated by other local factors – perhaps produced by stressing the bones in question, by mimicking the normal response to such stress, or even by exposing them briefly to some innocuous form of tissue-penetrating radiation. If the necessary activation procedures could not be readily repeated, the activated form of a pro-drug might also need to become attached to bone in its target area, so as to sustain the local effect.

LONG-ACTING BISPHOSPHONATE THERAPY?

Other types of non-hormonal drug therapy might also keep remodelling in balance for long periods. The existing bisphosphonates already go some way to satisfying the need. A longer-acting development of those currently available might bond even more persistently to bone mineral, inhibiting local osteoclast activity semi-permanently. But this may not be desirable – in view of the doubts already raised about the long-term quality of bone that is prevented from undergoing regular remodelling and rejuvenation. It may, therefore, be preferable to modify bisphosphonates in ways that avoid this possibility.

Suppose that an anabolic hormone could be bonded to the free end of a bisphosphonate molecule, leaving its characteristic P–C–P structure to become attached to hydroxyapatite in the usual way. If a combined bisphosphonate – anabolic molecule of this sort could also be targeted on fracture-prone areas of bone, such as the femoral neck in the elderly, local osteoclastic resorption might be inhibited while the local osteoblasts were stimulated to form new bone. But, however the future develops, today's innovations are sure to be superseded – as are tomorrow's in their turn. The idea of long-term therapy, built into the bones themselves to control the rates of both resorption and formation, may seem far-fetched today, but it could be taken further. If a future compound of this kind were bonded selectively to trabecular bone in the femoral neck or the bodies of the lumbar vertebrae, it might also be possible to regulate the local remodelling processes from outside the body.

RESTORING RUPTURED TRABECULAE?

If the medicine of the future seeks to exploit biological processes rather than work against them (many of today's drugs are prefixed '*anti-*' because they antagonize or block physiological activities), the normal mechanisms of fracture repair might be recruited to restore disrupted trabeculae. Fractures in osteoporotic bone heal as well as they do because the osteoclasts and osteoblasts, which clear the site, form callus and then remodel it into trabecular bone, perform these functions just as they would in normal bone. In doing so, they demonstrate that rarefied bone and ruptured trabeculae can be restored quite rapidly to greater strength and integrity.

It must be possible to exploit these unique reparative processes to restore the trabecular structure of osteoporotic bone – without having to fracture it first. Injection of a small amount of the patient's own blood into the crumbling trabeculae of an osteoporotic femoral neck or vertebral body, perhaps coupled with modest disturbance of its internal structure, might well have the desired effect of inducing local callus formation. The growth of new trabeculae could then be left to natural processes, perhaps aided by HRT or anabolic steroids to assist their development, plus calcium and vitamin D supplements to promote full mineralization, and followed by maintenance therapy to prevent subsequent resorption.

Pre-emptive pinning of a weak femoral neck – technically far simpler than after a fracture and very much less traumatic for the patient – might even be considered if its mineral density was low and the patient prone to fall. A conventional stainless steel pin should serve, but a coral pin of the type already in limited use for fracture repair – or similar ones made of synthetic coral or bone substitute – should not only

reinforce the femoral neck immediately but be gradually resorbed and replaced by living bone. More elegant ways of stimulating local regeneration may yet be found, but only if more research is devoted to the principle of inducing the body itself to rebuild, and then both retain and remodel, the strong trabecular framework that osteoporotic bone so conspicuously lacks.

CORRECTING GENETIC ABNORMALITIES

Finally, it should soon become possible to unravel some of the genetic mechanisms that appear to predispose to osteoporosis, whether by impairing the peak bone mass, by accelerating bone loss, or by both in succession. As the vast international research endeavor known as the Human Genome Project nears completion, its ambition of revealing the entire genetic constitution of human kind is bound to reveal countless anomalies. Every one of us is, after all, so different in detail as to be unique – though very like others. The exploration of the borders of normality, and the circumstances in which a few anomalous genes, not necessarily pathogenic in isolation, may conspire to cause or predispose to disease should be a fruitful field of research far into the future. The possible permutations and commutations are so astronomical in their number and complexity that they may never be fully analyzed. Research into them will therefore have to be target-oriented.

Genetic anomalies relevant to osteoporosis might be expected to affect the synthesis of bone collagen, of sex or other hormones, and of enzymes or transmitters concerned in calcium absorption and/or the mineralization of collagen matrix. Some might be severe enough to justify gene therapy, i.e. replacement of the anomalous gene or genes by normal ones. Since the search is already under way for the genetic faults responsible for the abnormal bone collagen in osteogenesis imperfecta (the congenital brittle bone disease, typically presenting in children), similar but less deleterious collagen defects predisposing to osteoporosis may also be identified within the next few years. If such defects led to bone matrix being deficient in quantity, faulty in structure, or perhaps less durable than normal, the affected bones would also be low in mineral density and consequently fracture prone. If genetic faults are found to impair the development of bone collagen in these ways, it might only be necessary to correct the more severe of them. Compensation could be made for minor anomalies by simpler means – calcium and vitamin D supplements, say, or hormone replacement. But the scope for future intervention seems certain to fly far higher …

More than any other field of research, genetics promises to open up a veritable Pandora's box of fantastic possibilities for modifying every aspect of the human form and probably much behavior, together with the structure and function of all plants and animals. From correction of genetic faults it would be but a short step to improving on nature. Far-fetched possibilities like implanting genes coding for stronger (African-type) bones in youth, for postmenopausal and younger amenorrheic women to synthesize their own HRT, or the elderly their own anabolic steroids could all become feasible in the future. The accumulation of minor genetic faults thought to underlie aging could perhaps be deferred or their effects prevented from weakening the bones in old age. We shall shortly be acquiring major keys to our own destiny – without practical instructions or ethical guidelines for their proper use. The prospects seem bright. It may, therefore, be salutary to reflect that the original Pandora's box of Greek mythology promised much but turned out to have contained all the ills of mankind, leaving only hope …

WHERE ARE WE GOING?

Modern scientific medicine is always travelling hopefully. It owes its many achievements to questioning assumptions, old and new, putting them to the test, and then challenging both the latest research findings and the conclusions based on them all over again. Science may travel hopefully but it never arrives – because it has no destination other than the pursuit of knowledge, wherever that may lead. In a complex condition like osteoporosis, which verges on normality and affects everybody to some degree over the course of a lifetime, medical research will come up with masses of detailed information, constantly being added to and revised, but not necessarily forming a coherent picture. Hence the numerous bits and pieces of half-baked medical advice about supposedly healthy diets and lifestyles, often based on incomplete research, with which the public is constantly regaled in ill-digested form.

The inevitable result is not a practical plan for healthier living, but confusion. Fortunately, in the field of osteoporosis (and a growing number of other disorders), so-called Consensus Conferences of leading specialists from different countries now produce concise professional guidelines, regularly updated. Invaluable though they are, these reports are not widely enough distributed to general practitioners and other clinicians, still less to patients, for their sensible, practical advice to be heeded or adopted on a scale commensurate with the problem. National osteoporosis societies are doing more than other bodies, professional or lay, to fill the gap by disseminating information and encouraging postmenopausal women in particular to seek medical advice and/or densitometry.

As doctors and patients become better informed, and the growing demand for densitometry makes screening facilities more widely available, it should become progressively easier to identify those at risk. But it will always be necessary to bear in mind that some may not want to know what is happening to their bones (or their blood pressure, or breasts or cervix for that matter), preferring to live their own lives and take the consequences. Medicine cannot claim the omnipotence, nor health 'authorities' the power, to overrule them. Most people do feel the need to take reasonable precautions, but it is no service to them to generate undue anxiety with semi-official health warnings, confusing advice, and questionable restrictions, however well-intentioned. Health guidance needs to be offered, persuasively, not forced down people's throats. It also needs to be simple, straightforward and, above all, well founded.

A recent American study identified 15 risk factors in the average outpatient, requiring a total of 25 interventions for their correction. Risk factors for osteoporosis were not among them, but that only serves to emphasize the point that people cannot be expected to go through life constantly looking over their shoulders – in case some dread disease is creeping up on them unawares. Much health education seems to have done more to generate guilt, anxiety and uncertainty than to prevent disease. Fussing about every risk factor that might pose a threat, or every prophylactic measure that purports to avert it, is no highroad to better health or happiness. None of us will live for ever, no matter what precautions we take.

Neither building a strong skeleton in youth nor taking preventive therapy later in life is likely to add appreciably to the average lifespan. But, as shown at the end of the previous chapter, there is a good chance of improving its quality – especially after the menopause and in old age – simply by reducing the risk of fractures and chronic disability. With that in mind, every child and adolescent ought to be given the opportunity to build strong bones. Every adult identifiably at risk – female or male, of any age – should be offered densitometry and given sufficient information and medical advice about their need for preventive therapy and what it entails to give each of us the choice – denied to all previous generations – of setting our own priorities and making our own well-informed decisions. Better understanding of osteoporosis is but the first step in just one increasingly challenging field of medicine.

Bibliographical notes

Foreseeable advances in drug therapy range from further development of current ideas [Heath D.A. (1993), Osteoporosis: current controversies and future trends, *Baillieres Clin. Rheumatol.*, **7**, 623–34; Brandi M.L. (1993), New treatment strategies: ipriflavone, strontium, vitamin D metabolites and analogs, *Am. J. Med.*, **95 suppl. 5A**, 69S–74S; Oursler M.J. *et al.* (1993), Echistatin, a potential new drug for osteoporosis (editorial), *Endocrinology*, **132**, 939–40] to novel concepts like the exploitation of selected actions of growth hormones after bone growth has ceased [Brixen K. *et al.* (1993), Growth hormone and adult bone remodeling: the potential use of GH in treatment of osteoporosis, *J. Pediat. Endocrinol.*, **6**, 65–71; Rosen C.J. *et al.* (1994), Insulin-like growth factors and bone: the osteoporosis connection, *Proc. Soc. Exp. Biol. Med.*, **206**, 83–102]. In the last chapter of his book *Bone remodeling and its disorders* [Martin Dunitz, London 1995, pp. 200–9], Gregory R. Mundy discusses (and references) many ideas for potential new treatments for osteoporosis. Two other papers also stimulate thought about the possible course of future progress [MacIntyre I. (1993), New perspectives in osteoporosis, *Trends Pharmacol. Sci.*, **14**, 319–20; Mundy G.R. (1993), Visions for the future in osteoporosis research, *Osteoporos. Int.*, **3 suppl. 2**, S29–34].

Glossary of technical terms

Underlined words refer to other entries

Adrenals: Pair of glands, on top of kidneys, each secreting adrenalin from internal medulla; corticosteroids and some sex hormones from surface cortex

Amenorrhea: Absence of menstruation, associated with ovarian failure, lack of ovulation and estradiol deficiency; underlying causes may lie in ovary (e.g. menopause), or act via hypothalamus or pituitary (e.g. anorexia, intensive exercise)

Amino acids: Nitrogen-containing building blocks of all proteins and peptides

Anabolic steroids: Synthetic analogues of testosterone, which build up bone, muscle and other tissues with less masculinization (in women)

Androgens: Male (literally 'man-making') sex hormones, notably testosterone and its metabolite, dihydrotestosterone

Androstenedione: Natural androgen, mainly secreted by adrenal cortex, much subsequently converted into estrogens

Anorexia nervosa: Eating disorder of unknown cause resulting in chronic self-starvation and often amenorrhea

Apatite: Shortened form of hydroxyapatite, the principal bone mineral

Bisphosphonates: Synthetic non-hormonal drugs, used for preventive therapy of osteoporosis, which act by inhibiting bone resorption; formerly known as diphosphonates

BMI: Body mass index

Body mass index: Index of nutritional state, which correlates well with body fat content; calculated by dividing weight (kg) by square of height (m²); low values associated with amenorrhea in anorexics, athletes, drug addicts, etc.

Bone biopsy: Surgical removal of bone sample, usually from iliac crest of pelvis, for microscopic examination and/or determination of mineral density

Bone density: The mineral density (i.e. calcium content) of bone, as measured by densitometry

Bone formation: The reconstruction phase of bone remodelling, particularly active during growth, fracture repair, and high bone turnover

Bone Gla protein: Osteocalcin, a minor non-collagenous component of normal bone matrix, used to measure bone formation

Bone loss: Decline in bone mass, usually measured in terms of mineral density, leading to osteoporosis if resorption too rapid or prolonged for bone formation to keep pace

Bone mass: The total amount of bone matrix and bone mineral at a particular site or in the whole body

Bone matrix: The mainly collagen framework which gives bones their shape and provides the resilient structure on which bone mineral is laid down

Bone mineral: Mainly hydroxyapatite, deposited on the bone matrix to give bones their hardness and strength

Bone mineral content: The quantity of mineral present in a given area of bone, as measured by densitometry

Bone remodelling: Process of constant renewal: resorption of old bone by osteoclasts and its regeneration by osteoblasts

Bone resorption: Breaking down and removal of both bone mineral and bone matrix by osteoclasts

Bone turnover: The rate at which remodelling replaces old bone with new; raised following estrogen withdrawal, particularly after menopause or withdrawal of HRT

Brittle-bone disease: Popular term for conditions in which pathological fractures occur, chiefly osteogenesis imperfecta in children and osteoporosis in adults

Bulimia: Compulsive eating disorder of unknown cause, related to anorexia nervosa, with bouts of gorging followed by deliberate or involuntary vomiting, typically resulting in weight loss and amenorrhea

Calciferol: Vitamin D, a mixture of related compounds, chiefly ergocalciferol (vit. D$_2$) and cholecalciferol (vit. D$_3$)

Calcification: Abnormal deposition of calcium salts in soft tissues; distinguish from normal mineralization of bone

Calcitonin: Peptide hormone secreted by C-cells of thyroid, also obtained from pig and salmon, sniffed up or injected in synthetic form as preventive therapy for osteoporosis, to reduce bone resorption

Calcitriol: 1,25 dihydroxy-cholecalciferol, an active metabolite of vitamin D, responsible for much of its effect on bone

Calcium balance: The prevailing balance between calcium absorption and excretion, normally positive until peak bone mass, negative thereafter – especially after menopause, in old age, and in patients with osteoporotic bone loss

Calcium requirements: The total daily intake of calcium (from diet and supplements) required to keep the body in calcium balance, after allowing for poor absorption and the prevailing rate of excretion

Calcium salts: Principal constituents of bone mineral, chiefly obtained from milk and milk products

Callus: Poorly structured bone formed around fracture sites as the first stage of regeneration, then remodelled into trabecular and/or cortical bone

Cancellous bone: Synonym for trabecular or 'spongy' bone

Cartilage: Firm elastic tissue of several types, composed of collagen and proteoglycans; smooth-surfaced hyaline type covers the bone ends in synovial joints

Cervix (uteri): The neck of the womb, opening downwards into the vagina

Collagen: Structural protein of several types (literally 'glue-forming' because converted to gelatin by boiling); commonest tissue in the body, main component of bone matrix (type I collagen) and cartilage

Collagen breakdown products: Metabolites (e.g. hydroxyproline, cross-links), measured to determine rate and/or balance of bone remodelling

Colles' fracture: Fracture of forearm bones (radius and ulna) just above wrist, common in menopausal women, suggestive of osteoporosis

Combipatch: Popular term for Estracombi skin patch; form of transdermal HRT combining estradiol and progestogen

Compact bone: Synonym for cortical bone

Computer tomography: Computerized X-ray imaging technique displaying internal body structures in layers; quantifiable for use as densitometry

Conjugated estrogens: Mixed sodium salts of the sulfate esters of estrogens, marketed as Premarin

Corpus luteum: 'Yellow body' that develops in ruptured ovarian follicle, following ovulation, and secretes progesterone during luteal phase of menstrual cycle (and in pregnancy)

Cortex: Surface layer of adrenals, cortical bone, brain, etc.

Cortical bone: Dense bone, mainly forming the tubular shafts of long bones; less affected by osteoporosis, until old age, than trabecular bone

Corticosteroids: Steroid hormones normally secreted by adrenal cortex, but an important cause of osteoporotic bone loss when synthesized for use as long-term drug treatment

Cross-links: Fragments of type I collagen, specifically from bone matrix; estimation of their urinary excretion rate reflects rate of bone resorption

CT: Computer tomography

Densitometry: Measurement of bone density by various methods, preferably dual-energy X-ray absorptiometry

DXA: Dual-energy X-ray absorptiometry

Dihydrotestosterone: Active metabolite of testosterone, helps to protect against osteoporosis, but responsible for stimulating prostatic enlargement with age

Diphosphonates: Now known as bisphosphonates

DPA: Dual-photon absorptiometry

Dual-energy X-ray absorptiometry: Most widely applicable and versatile densitometry technique for forearm, hip, spine, including lateral views

Dual-photon absorptiometry: Versatile densitometry technique, being superseded by DXA

Dyspareunia: Pain, usually in vagina, on sexual intercourse, commonly caused by estradiol deficiency following menopause

Embryo: The developing fertilized ovum up to the beginning of the 3rd month of human pregnancy, when all the organs, limbs, etc. have been differentiated – to form a fetus

Endocrine gland: Any organ synthesizing and/or secreting an endocrine hormone

Endocrine hormones: Chemical messengers secreted into the bloodstream to act elsewhere in the body, including all pituitary and sex hormones, insulin, thyroid and parathyroid hormones, adrenalin and corticosteroids secreted by adrenals

Endometrium: Lining layer of uterus, responsive to estrogens and progesterone, discarded during menstruation

Equilin: Non-human estrogen from pregnant mares, present in Premarin

Estracombi: Transdermal HRT in form of skin patches containing estradiol combined with the progestogen, norethisterone

Estraderm: Transdermal patches containing natural estradiol for application to, and absorption through, the skin

Estradiol: Natural estrogen secreted by ovarian follicles from menarche to menopause, deficient thereafter; various forms given in HRT to treat hot flushes and other acute menopausal symptoms, long-term to prevent osteoporosis and cardiovascular disease

Estriol: Relatively weak estrogen with little effect on bone density, endometrium or other tissues, formed by reduction of estrone and estradiol; freely excreted in urine

Estrogens: Female steroidal sex hormones (literally 'estrus-making', i.e. promoting fertile phase), the three main ones named after the number of hydroxy (OH) groups in their steroid molecules: estrone, estradiol, estriol

Estrogen deficiency: Lack of (mainly) estradiol, in amenorrhea and after the menopause

Estrogen implants: Form of HRT, usually consisting of estradiol pellets for subcutaneous insertion every 4–6 months

Estrone: Estrogen, weaker oxidation product of estradiol, more active than estriol; some secreted by ovaries, most converted peripherally (in body fat, etc.) from estradiol and from the androgen, androstenedione

Estrus: Regular fertile spells in female mammals ('on heat'), coinciding with ovulation

Fallopian tubes: Paired passages linking each ovary to the uterus, enabling the ovum to reach the uterine cavity

Femur: Thigh bone; fracture of neck or upper shaft common in old age; femoral neck commonly used for densitometry

Fertilization: Union of sperm with ovum, leading to formation of the embryo

Fetus: The fully formed embryo growing from early in the 3rd month of pregnancy to birth

First-pass effect: Metabolic modification of anything taken by mouth (drugs, nutrients, food additives, etc.), which must first pass through the liver after absorption

Fluorides: Fluorine compounds which strengthen teeth and, in larger amounts, promote formation of woven bone; excess causes fluorosis

Fluorosis: Pathological condition, mainly of skeleton, caused by excessive fluoride intake, consisting of osteosclerosis with some osteomalacia

Follicles: Potential ovum-producing cells in the ovaries

Follicle stimulating hormone: Pituitary hormone which stimulates growth of Graafian follicle in ovary and secretion of estradiol during follicular phase of menstrual cycle. Also initiates puberty and stimulates testosterone secretion in the male

Follicular phase: First half of menstrual cycle, in which developing follicle secretes estradiol, culminating in ovulation

Follicular rupture: The mechanism of ovulation

Fracture threshold: The notional level of bone density below which bones become prone to pathological fractures

FSH: Follicle stimulating hormone

GH: <u>Growth hormone</u>

Gametes: Haploid reproductive cells (i.e. with a single set of chromosomes): <u>ovum</u> in females, <u>spermatozoa</u> in males

Gestagens: Natural or synthetic hormones with <u>progestogenic</u> activity

GnRH: <u>Gonadotropin releasing hormone</u>

Gonadotropins: <u>FSH</u> and <u>LH</u> secreted by <u>pituitary</u> to stimulate <u>sex hormone</u> secretion by the male and female <u>gonads</u>

Gonadotropin releasing hormone: Locally acting hormone secreted by <u>hypothalamus</u>, to stimulate secretion of <u>gonadotropins</u> by adjacent <u>pituitary</u>

Gonads: <u>Gamete</u>- and <u>sex-hormone</u>-producing reproductive glands of either sex: <u>ovaries</u> in females, <u>testes</u> in males

Graafian follicle: <u>Ovarian follicle</u> which develops during <u>follicular phase</u> of <u>menstrual cycle</u>; first described by Netherlands' anatomist, Reinier de Graaf (1641–73)

Greenstick fracture: A bend rather than an actual break in pliable, poorly mineralized bone, usually in children

Growth hormone: <u>Pituitary hormone</u> which stimulates (bone) growth through-out childhood, notably in conjunction with <u>sex hormones</u> at <u>puberty</u>

Hormone: Biochemical messenger or <u>mediator</u>, usually produced by an <u>endocrine gland</u>, to act elsewhere in the body

Hormone replacement therapy: Any <u>hormone</u> given to replace a deficient one, usually applied to <u>estrogen</u>/<u>progestogen</u> replacement after the <u>menopause</u>

Hot flushes: Prominent symptom of <u>estrogen withdrawal</u>, especially at <u>menopause</u>, affecting less than 50% of women

HRT: <u>Hormone replacement therapy</u>

Hyaline cartilage: Smooth-surfaced lining of <u>synovial joints</u>

Hydroxyapatite: <u>Bone mineral</u>, mainly <u>calcium phosphate</u>

Hydroxyproline: <u>Metabolite</u> of all types of <u>collagen</u>; excretion rate gives measure of <u>collagen</u> turnover, but not specific to <u>bone matrix</u>

Hypothalamus: Small area in base of brain just above <u>pituitary</u>; responsible for stimulating onset of <u>puberty</u> and governing <u>menstrual cycle</u>

Hysterectomy: Surgical removal of <u>uterus</u>, together with ('total' hysterectomy) or without the <u>ovaries</u>

Induced menopause: Artificial <u>premature menopause</u>, resulting from <u>ovariectomy</u> or exposure of <u>ovaries</u> to chemotherapy or irradiation

Introitus: The <u>vulva</u> or entrance to the <u>vagina</u>

LH: <u>Luteinizing hormone</u>

Libido: Sexual drive (literally: desire, lust) in either sex, though used more of females

Lining cells: Modified <u>osteocytes</u> lining spaces in <u>trabecular</u> bone

Luteal phase: Second half of <u>menstrual cycle</u>, following <u>ovulation</u>, in which <u>corpus luteum</u> secretes <u>progesterone</u>

Luteinizing hormone: <u>Pituitary</u> hormone which promotes <u>luteal phase</u> and stimulates <u>progesterone secretion</u> by <u>corpus luteum</u>; also, with <u>FSH</u>, stimulates <u>puberty</u> in both sexes

Magnetic resonance imaging: Non-invasive method of visualizing internal organs and structures without X-rays

Masculinization: The production of male-type secondary sexual characteristics, usually in females

Mediators: Body chemicals released by a cell, or part of it, in response to a stimulus, to act on another cell, or part of it; see paracrine hormones

Menarche: Time of first menstruation

Menopausal symptoms: Hot flushes, palpitations, psychological disturbance, dyspareunia, pruritus vulvae, loss of libido, increased frequency and/or pain on passing urine – all caused by estrogen withdrawal but differing widely in severity

Menopause: Permanent cessation (not 'pause') of menstruation at any age, normally between 45 and 55, when ovaries run out of follicles and can no longer respond to stimulation by the pituitary hormones FSH and LH; therefore associated with estrogen (and progesterone) deficiency

Menstrual cycle: Regular cycle of menstrual (literally 'monthly') bleeding and ovulation

Menstruation: Menstrual bleeding, with loss of endometrium

Metacarpal index: Simplest form of X-ray densitometry, in middle metacarpal bone of hand, which relates total thickness of cortex to overall diameter, both in mid-shaft

Metabolite: Any compound resulting from biochemical modification or breakdown of another (whether from outside, e.g. drug or pollutant, or a hormone or other body constituent); may be biologically active or inert

MI: Metacarpal index

Mineral density: Calcium content of bone, as measured by densitometry

Mineralization: Process of laying down bone mineral on the bone matrix

MRI: Magnetic resonance imaging

Oligomenorrhea: Scanty and/or very occasional menstruation

Oophorectomy: Surgical removal of one or (usually) both ovaries, on their own or as part of total hysterectomy; invariably precipitates premature menopause and estrogen deficiency in a woman of childbearing age

Osteoblasts: Bone-forming cells responsible for building bone matrix and its mineralization, at remodelling sites

Osteocalcin: Bone Gla protein, a minor non-collagenous structural component of normal bone matrix, used as a measure of bone formation

Osteoclasts: Larger, multinucleated cells responsible for bone resorption, clearing remodelling sites for new bone formation

Osteocytes: Resident cells scattered throughout bone, probably overseeing its day-to-day metabolism and longer-term remodelling

Osteogenesis imperfecta: Inherited anomaly, in which bone matrix is genetically defective, with predisposition to fractures

Osteoid: Bone matrix that has not been mineralized

Osteomalacia: Adult counterpart of rickets, in which bone matrix is undermineralized, caused by deficiency of vitamin D (and dietary calcium). May coexist with osteoporosis

Osteopenia: Deficiency in quantity of bone, both matrix and mineral, especially <u>osteoporosis</u>

Osteoporosis: Condition resulting from loss of bone, both <u>matrix</u> and <u>mineral</u>, with predisposition to fractures, caused mainly by <u>sex hormone</u> deficiency, especially after the menopause (<u>type I</u>), and in old age (<u>type II</u>). May coexist with <u>osteomalacia</u>

Osteosclerosis: Pathologically increased <u>density</u> of bone

Ovarian follicles: Primordial cells present in <u>ovaries</u> before birth, one of which typically develops into a <u>Graafian follicle</u> about the middle of each non-pregnant month, from soon after <u>menarche</u> to <u>menopause</u>

Ovariectomy: Same as <u>oophorectomy</u>: removal of one or both <u>ovaries</u>, precipitating <u>menopause</u> and <u>estrogen deficiency</u>

Ovaries: Female <u>gonads</u>, one on each side of uterus, containing <u>follicles</u> responsible for <u>ovulation</u> and for secretion of <u>estrogens</u> and <u>progesterone</u>

Ovulation: Release of egg or <u>ovum</u> from ruptured <u>Graafian follicle</u> about half-way through <u>menstrual cycle</u>

Ovum: The unfertilized female egg released at <u>ovulation</u>

Paracrine: Refers to the action of <u>hormones</u> or <u>mediators</u> produced locally by <u>endocrine glands</u> or other cells

Parathyroid: Small glands alongside thyroid which secrete <u>parathyroid hormone</u> (<u>PTH</u>)

Parathyroid hormone: Natural <u>hormone</u>, secreted by <u>parathyroids</u>, which promotes bone <u>resorption</u>

Parenteral: Other than by mouth, used to describe drugs given by injection, infusion, inhalation, skin application, etc.

Pathological fracture: Any fracture to which bone disease, such as <u>osteoporosis</u>, has predisposed

Peak bone mass: The maximum amount of bone actually attained by an individual, usually by the age of 30 – a valuable concept put to little practical use, because rarely measured

Peptide hormones: Non-steroid hormones of protein structure, digested if taken by mouth, e.g. <u>calcitonin</u>, which have to be taken <u>parenterally</u>

Perimenopausal: Refers to the period of months or years around the <u>menopause</u>

Periosteum: Tough surface membrane of all bones, actively concerned in growth, surface <u>remodelling</u>, and repair

Pituitary: <u>Endocrine gland</u> at base of brain with distinct anterior and posterior parts; described as 'conductor of the endocrine orchestra' because it secretes a broad range of control <u>hormones</u> which regulate all endocrine activity throughout the body, including growth, <u>puberty</u> and <u>menstruation</u>, but not the <u>menopause</u>

Pituitary hormones: Range of control hormones (e.g. <u>growth hormone</u>, <u>follicle stimulating hormone</u>, <u>luteinizing hormone</u>) secreted by <u>pituitary</u>

Postmenopausal: To do with period following <u>menopause</u>, usually refers to first few years though applicable to rest of life

Premarin: <u>Conjugated estrogens</u> extracted from pregnant mares' urine, containing 17α-<u>estradiol</u>, sodium <u>estrone</u> sulfate, and <u>equilin</u>

Premenopausal: To do with period of months or years leading up to <u>menopause</u>

Progesterone: <u>Steroid hormone</u> (literally 'favoring gestation', i.e. pregnancy) normally secreted by <u>corpus luteum</u> during <u>luteal phase</u> of <u>menstrual cycle</u>

Progestin: Originally, the first crude extracts of <u>corpus luteum</u> found to have progestational activity; now often used for natural or synthetic hormones with similar actions, i.e. <u>gestagens</u>, <u>progestogens</u>

Progestogen: Synthetic <u>hormone</u> with <u>progesterone</u>-like activity

Progestogenic: Acting like <u>progesterone</u>

Pruritus vulvae: Itching irritation in <u>vulva</u> (and/or <u>vagina</u>)

PTH: <u>Parathyroid hormone</u>

Puberty: The period of sexual development and rapid growth that normally marks the onset of adolescence

QCT: Quantitative <u>computer tomography</u>, used as a form of <u>densitometry</u>

Radius: Forearm bone commonly fractured in menopausal women, used for <u>densitometry</u>

Regeneration: Self-repair or replacement of tissue without scarring, restricted in mammals to bone and liver

Remodelling: Process of constant <u>resorption</u> of old bone by <u>osteoclasts</u> and its <u>regeneration</u> by <u>osteoblasts</u>

Remodelling sites: Parts of bone in which <u>remodelling</u> is active

Resorption: Breaking down and removal of both <u>bone mineral</u> and <u>bone matrix</u> by <u>osteoclasts</u>

Rickets: Maldevelopment of skeleton in children caused by lack of <u>vitamin D</u> and <u>calcium</u>. Childhood counterpart of <u>osteomalacia</u>

Secondary sexual characteristics: Features typical of adolescent/adult male (facial and pubic hair, deepening of voice, muscularity, etc.) or female (breast development, pubic hair, figure, etc.) induced by <u>androgens</u> and <u>estrogens</u>, respectively, at puberty or in later response to <u>sex hormone</u> therapy

Sex hormones: <u>Endocrine hormones</u> regulating sexual development and functions, notably <u>estrogens</u> and <u>progesterone</u> in females, <u>testosterone</u> in males. Also, <u>control hormones</u>: <u>GnRH</u>, <u>FSH</u>, and <u>LH</u>

Sex steroids: <u>Sex hormones</u> with a <u>steroid</u> structure

Single-photon absorptiometry: <u>Densitometry</u> technique applicable to forearm bones, not hip or spine; possible screening test for <u>osteoporosis</u>

SPA: <u>Single-photon absorptiometry</u>

Spermatozoa: Male <u>gametes</u> produced by <u>testes</u>

Spongy bone: Synonym for <u>trabecular</u> or <u>cancellous</u> bone

Steroid hormones: All hormones with steroidal structure

Subcutaneous implants: Drug or <u>hormone</u> pellets (especially of <u>estradiol</u> or <u>testosterone</u>) inserted under skin at intervals of many months for gradual release, as long-term treatment or <u>hormone replacement</u>

Synovial joints: All free-moving joints between bones, notably in limbs, lined with smooth synovial membrane and lubricated by synovial fluid

Testes: Male <u>gonads</u>, producing <u>spermatozoa</u> and secreting <u>testosterone</u>, located in scrotum for optimal functioning below body temperature

Testosterone: Male steroid sex hormone, responsible for reproductive functions and virility; maintains bone strength by keeping remodelling in balance

Tibolone: Synthetic steroid with weak estrogenic, androgenic and progestogenic properties, used as HRT without stimulating endometrium or causing menstruation

Trabecular bone: Bone with open lattice-work structure, combining lightness with strength, at ends of long bones, in vertebral bodies and in pelvis, scapula, etc.; frequently remodelled and more prone to osteoporosis than cortical bone

Transdermal administration: Way of giving systemic hormone or drug treatment by absorption through the skin from adhesive patches, commonly used for HRT with estradiol, testosterone, progestogen, etc.

TTS: Transdermal therapeutic system, or skin patch (e.g. Estraderm), for controlled absorption of drug through skin

Type I osteoporosis: Typically postmenopausal; caused by estrogen deficiency in women, testosterone deficiency in men

Type II osteoporosis: Also known as 'senile', associated with aging in either sex

Uterus: Anatomical term for the womb, including its hollow body, muscular walls, lining endometrium, and cervix

Vertebral body: The large weight-bearing drum in each vertebra, consisting mainly of trabecular bone; particularly prone to osteoporosis and fracture in recently menopausal women

Virilization: Production of male characteristics by androgens

Virilism: Abnormal development of male characteristics in females

Virility: Male vigor, sexual potency

Vitamin D: Mixed vitamin (see calciferol) present in fish liver oils, dairy products, etc., also synthesized from sterols in skin on exposure to ultra-violet light; normally promotes calcium absorption and mineralization of bone; deficiency causes rickets and osteomalacia; excess also harmful

Vagina: The 'front passage' linking vulva and uterus

Vulva: The entrance or introitus to the vagina

Ward's triangle: Triangular area of bone in neck of femur

Woven bone: Bone of low strength with poorly oriented collagen fibers in its matrix; normal in embryo and young children; also formed in adults treated with fluoride salts and in cases of fluorosis

Sources of illustrations

The author and Publishers would like to acknowledge with thanks the following permissions that have kindly been granted by authors and publishers for the use of material in this publication. Every effort has been made to contact holders of copyright to obtain permission to reproduce copyright material. However, if any have been inadvertently overlooked, the publishers will be pleased to make the necessary arrangements at the first opportunity.

The following figures and tables have been reproduced or adapted from Leif Mosekilde: *Knoglevævets Biologi*, ISBN 87-983055-14, with permission: **Chapter 1**: *Figures 3a, 3b, 8*; **Chapter 2**: *Figures 3a, 3b, 4a, 4b, 5, 6, 7, 8, 11b*; **Chapter 3**: *Figure 9*; **Chapter 6**: *Figures 3a, 3b, 3c*

The following figures have been reproduced from Aarhus Bone and Mineral Research Group, with permission: **Chapter 4**: *Figure 10*; **Chapter 5**: *Figure 7*; **Chapter 6**: *Figures 2a, 2b, 2c, 20*

The following figures and tables by the late Frank Netter have been reproduced from the *Ciba Collection of Medical Illustrations* or *Clinical Symposia* with permission of Ciba-Geigy: **Chapter 1**: *Figures 1, 2a, 2b, 4, 6, 7, 9 and Table 1*; **Chapter 2**: *Figures 2, 9, 10, 11a*; **Chapter 3**: *Figures 2, 6, 7, 8, 12*; **Chapter 4**: *Figure 2*; **Chapter 5**: *Figures 2a, 2b, 3, 4, 9, 11, 14, 15*; **Chapter 6**: *Figures 23, 27, 29*

Permissions kindly granted for individual figures are as follows:

Chapter 1

Figure 10 Kluwer Academic Publishers, Lancaster, England, from Cope, E. (1976). In Campbell, S. (ed.) *The Management of the Menopausal and Postmenopausal Years*. (Lancaster: MTP Press)

Figure 11 Annals of Internal Medicine, American College of Physicians from Kannel, W.B. (1976). Menopause and risk of cardiovascular disease; the Framingham Study. *Ann. Intern. Med.*, **85**, 407–502

Figure 12 Christiansen, C. *et al.* (1981). Bone mass in postmenopausal women after withdrawal of oestrogen/gestagen replacement therapy. *Lancet*, **1**, 459–61. © The Lancet Ltd.

Chapter 2

Figure 12 The National Dairy Council

Figure 14 Chris Priest and Mark Clarke / Science Photo Library

Chapter 3

Figure 3 Churchill Livingstone, from Fink, G. (1979). *Br. Med. Bull.*, **35**, 155

Figure 5 The Johns Hopkins University School of Hygiene and Public Health from Willett, W. *et al.* (1983). Cigarette smoking, relative weight, and menopause. *Am. J. Epidemiol.*, **117**, 651–8

Figures 10 and 11 Gosden, R.G. (1985). *Biology of Menopause.* (Orlando, London: Academic Press)

Chapter 4

Figures 3 and 4 With permission, J. Gill/CGSP

Figure 5 Department of Rheumatology, Wexham Park Hospital, Slough, UK

Figure 6 *Diet and Health: Implications for Reducing Chronic Risk.* © 1989. The National Academy of Sciences. Courtesy of the National Academy Press, Washington, DC

Figure 7 Christiansen, C. *et al.* (1981). Bone mass in postmenopausal women after withdrawal of oestrogen/gestagen replacement therapy. *Lancet*, **1**, 459–61. © The Lancet Ltd.

Figure 9 National Osteoporosis Society

Figure 11 BUPA

Chapter 5

Figure 1 Remy Poinot/Robert Harding Picture Library

Figure 8 Raven Press, from Riggs, B.L. and Melton, L.J., III (1988). *Osteoporosis – Etiology, Diagnosis and Management*, p. 235

Figure 10 Schlenker, R.A. and VonSeggen, W.W. (1976). The distribution of cortical and trabecular bone mass along the lengths of the radius and ulna, and the implications for *in vivo* bone mass measurements. *Calcified Tissue Res.*, **20**, 41–52. © Springer Verlag

Figures 12 and 13 Hologic Inc. and Vertec Scientific Ltd.

Chapter 6

Figures 4b and 7 Ribot, C. *et al.* (1989). Preventive effects of transdermal administration of 17β-estradiol on postmenopausal bone loss: a two year

prospective study. *Gynecol. Endocrinol.*, **3**, 259–67

Figure 4c Briancon, D. and Meunier, P.J. (1980). Le fluor en pathologie et en therapeutique osseuses. Son application au tratement des osteoporoses. *Lyon Med.*, **243**, 183–94

Figure 5 Fromm, G.A. (1991). Differential action of pamidronate on trabecular and cortical bone in women with involutional osteoporosis. *Osteoporosis Int.*, **1**, 129–33. © Springer Verlag

Figure 6 *Western Journal of Medicine*, from Riggs, B.L. (1991). Overview of osteoporosis. *Western J. Med.*, **154**, 63–77

Figure 11a Adapted from Advanced Drug Delivery Systems, Alza Corporation and Ciba-Geigy, 1976

Figure 11b Walsh, B. (1988). Relief of menopause symptoms by transdermal estradiol. In Birdwood, G. (ed.) *Transdermal Estrogen Replacement Therapy for Menopausal Women*, pp.29–34. (Berne: Hans Huber)

Figure 13 Whitehead, M.I. (1990). The development of transdermal estradiol therapy. In Whitehead, M.I. and Schenkel, L. (eds.) *Transdermal Hormone Replacement Therapy: Long-term Effects*, pp. 13–22. (Carnforth, UK: Parthenon Publishing)

Figure 14 Stevenson, J.C., Cust, M.P., Gangar, K.F., Hillard, T.C., Lees, B. and Whitehead, M.I. (1990). Effects of transdermal versus oral hormone replacement therapy on bone density in spine and proximal femur in postmenopausal women. *Lancet*, **336**, 265–9. © The Lancet Ltd

Figure 16a S. Karger AG, Basel, from Kanis, J.A. and McCloskey, E.V. (1990). The use of clodronate in disorders of calcium and skeletal metabolism. *Clinical Metabolism.* Volume 4 of *Progress in Basic Clinical Pharmacology*, pp. 89–136. (Basel: Karger)

Figures 16b and 16c Storm, T. *et al.*
(1990). Effect of intermittent cyclical
etidronate therapy on bone mass and
fracture rate in women with
postmenopausal osteoporosis. *N. Engl. J.
Med.*, **322**, 1265–71

Figure 17a Reginster, J.Y. *et al.* (1987).
1-year controlled randomised trial of
prevention of early postmenopausal
bone loss by intranasal calcitonin.
Lancet, **2**, 1481–3. © The Lancet Ltd.

Figure 17b BMJ Publishing Group, from
Overgaard, K. *et al.* (1989). Effect of
calcitonin given intranasally on early
postmenopausal bone loss. *Br. Med. J.*,
299, 477–9

Figure 18a Chesnut, C.H., III (1983).
Stanozolol in postmenopausal
osteoporosis: therapeutic efficacy and
possible mechanism(s) of action.
Metabolism, **32**, 571–80

Figure 18b Need, A.G. *et al.* (1983).
Effects of nandrolone decanoate and
antiresorptive therapy on vertebral
density in osteoporotic postmenopausal
women. *Arch. Intern. Med.*, **149**, 57–60.
© 1983, American Medical Association

Figures 19a–c Riggs, B.L. *et al.* (1990).
Effect of fluoride treatment on the
fracture rate in postmenopausal women
with osteoporosis. *N. Engl. J. Med.*, **322**,
802–9. Massachusetts Medical Society.
All rights reserved

Figure 21 BMJ Publishing Group.
Drawn from data in Chaupy, M.C.

et al. (1994). Effect of calcium and
cholecalciferal treatment for three years
in hip fractures in elderly women.
Br. Med. J., **308**, 1081–2

Figure 22 Smith, W.S. and Kaufer, H.
(1969). Patterns and mechanisms of
lumbar injuries associated with lap seat
belts. *J. Bone Joint Surg.*, **51A**, 239–54

Figure 24 Fink, G. (1979). *Br. Med.
Bull.*, **35**, 155

Figure 25b Staland, B. Continuous
treatment with a combination of
estrogen and gestagen – a way of
avoiding endometrial stimulation. *Acta
Obstet. Gynecol. Scand.*, **130** (Suppl.),
29–35

Figure 25c Schenkel, L. (1990).
Development of a combined
norethisterone acetate/estradiol TTS. In
Whitehead, M.I. and Schenkel, L. (eds.)
*Transdermal Hormone Replacement:
Long-term Effects.* (Carnforth, UK:
Parthenon Publishing)

Figure 26 Lindsay, R. *et al.* (1987).
Inter-relationship of bone loss and its
prevention, and fracture expression.
In Christiansen, C. *et al.* (eds.)
Osteoporosis, pp. 508–12.
(Copenhagen: Osteopress)

Table 7 Cummings, S.R. (1991).
Benefits and risks of long-term
postmenopausal hormone therapy.
In Samsioe, G. (ed.) *Cardiovascular
Disease and HRT – New Perspectives.*
(Carnforth, UK: Parthenon Publishing)

Index